WITH PEN IN HAND

The Healing Power of Writing

HENRIETTE ANNE KLAUSER

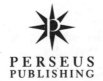

PERSEUS
PUBLISHING

A Member of the Perseus Books Group
Cambridge, Massachusetts

Cataloging-in-Publication Data is available from the Library of Congress.
ISBN 0–7382–0788–8

Perseus Publishing is a Member of the Perseus Books Group.

Find us on the World Wide Web at http://www.perseuspublishing.com

Perseus Publishing books are available at special discounts for bulk purchases in the United States by corporations, institutions, and other organizations. For more information, please contact the Special Markets Department at the Perseus Books Group, 11 Cambridge Center, Cambridge, MA 02142, or call (800) 255–1514 or (617) 252–5298, or e-mail j.mccrary@perseusbooks.com.

Text design by Trish Wilkinson
Set in 11.5-point Stempel Garamond by the Perseus Books Group

First printing, December 2002

1 2 3 4 5 6 7 8 9 10—06 05 04 03 02

To Grace Elizabeth and Maxwell Alexander
for the joy you bring me and for your
daily reminder of what matters
just by being you

Contents

Introduction

I was in Oklahoma City to give a presentation two weeks after Timothy McVeigh blew the Federal Building to smithereens, taking the lives of 168 people, 19 of them children. The Murrah Building wasn't the only thing McVeigh bombed; his cowardly act shattered the security of a nation for the first time, especially the ones most directly involved, the friends and relatives of those killed in the blast.

When I saw the sadness in the eyes of the audience in front of me, I threw away my prepared script and instead led 250 people through an exercise in writing about their misery.

Later, they sent me tender letters describing the effect. One such said simply, "Thank you for helping us put our hearts on paper, and in the process heal the broken parts."

My experience in Oklahoma is an example of healing writing at its best. This kind of writing is not about producing something polished and professional; it's about the power of the written word to soothe our souls and ease the anguish.

The poet W. S. Merwin was commissioned by *The New Yorker* to write about the disaster of September 11th. He said, "In moments of great grief or loss, we turn to words" to say "what cannot be said."

Four days after that attack, I was part of a therapeutic writing workshop. It was a chance, in a group, to sort through the horror and the confusion we all felt. We took our sadness and our rage and put it on the page where it could not harm us or anybody else. As we expressed our deepest feelings without reserve in poetry and prose, we felt the power of our words begin to draw out some of the pain from our hearts and replace it with hope.

With Pen in Hand: The Healing Power of Writing is a book that tells how to employ in times of great stress a simple tool available to all of us. It teaches this through a series of stories of people who were in trouble or in grief and needed help. They turned to writing as to a friend, to walk with them through the dark night.

With Pen in Hand deals with those times when you have to throw out the blueprint you had for your life and build from the ground up. Divorce. Death. Serious sickness. Abuse. Loss of job. Violence. Yes, even acts of terrorism. Life's disappointments and numbing tragedies are curveballs that hit us right in the face. Now what do you do? How do you go on living when your world has collapsed? And what do you do about the ache in your chest?

These pages present the true tales of people in pain, with this connecting thread: All of them used writing as a way to pick up the pieces and make them whole again.

Writing goes right to the place that hurts, and writing heals.

WHO AM I?

Let me introduce myself and tell you some of my background so you will know how I came to write this book. I have a Ph.D. in English literature and have taught at universities in New York, Los Angeles, Seattle, and Lethbridge, Canada, in Alberta. For the past 17 years, I have been giving workshops for corporations around the country and presentations at national associations. Internationally, I have conducted workshops in Greece, England, and Egypt. Perhaps you are familiar with my first book, *Writing on Both Sides of the Brain: Breakthrough Techniques for People Who Write.* It has been around for a long time. *Writing on Both Sides of the Brain* addresses the subject of writing anxiety. It is for people who have to write, and hate to write. It deals with procrastination and writer's block, and teaches how to separate the writing from the editing. I didn't know it at the time I was writing it, but there is a lot in there that applies to writing and healing.

My books grow out of what my readers tell me they want. It was my readers who said, after *Writing on Both Sides of the Brain,* "This isn't about writing; it's about life."

Then they proceeded to tell me how they were using writing to build relationship—the stories that led to my second book, *Put Your Heart on Paper: Staying Connected in a Loose-ends World.*

My third book, *Write It Down, Make It Happen,* started out as a single chapter in *Put Your Heart on Paper* and was expanded by the examples people sent me of dreams coming true.

Write It Down, Make It Happen is about goal setting, about events and successes outside of us. It tells how to pay attention to the signs and signals that you are on the right path and how to handle breakdown. The subtitle is *Knowing What You Want, and Getting It.*

All of my work centers around writing, that powerful tool to communicate that we learned in the first grade; now, to what nobler use could it be put than to heal a broken heart?

With Pen in Hand began with that workshop in Oklahoma, and was broadened by the mail I have received from all over the world sent to me from hurting people who have found solace in the salve of personal writing.

THE MAIL THAT
COMES FROM READERS

I see it over and over in the letters I get, from people who have read my books, and those I meet in the workshops I give. I am touched by the open way that people share their lives with me. The correspondence comes from all over the United States, from France and England, Scotland, Ireland, Romania, Turkey, Kuwait, Australia, New Zealand, Italy. Sometimes the English is halting, but no matter what the nationality, the courage and caring resound. Their letters are a testimonial to the difference writing makes.

Here are just a few examples.

- Marco went to the top of the mountain to meditate when his wife left him and his two little children. He had never tried writing before, but he was desperate for clues and answers to his terrible situation. He filled 30 pages on both sides, and told me, "I was so astonished,

I couldn't believe it; everything in my life began to change."

- When Bette's son was murdered, randomly killed by gunshot in Las Vegas, she told me she would have gone mad from the loss without writing to ground her.

- Dawn poured her heart out in unsent letters to her son who was abducted into a cult for two years. Those letters lifted some of the weight of her guilt and sorrow. She had no address to send them to, but the letter writing was "a conversation I desperately needed, even if my son could not hear my words."

- Hadifa Al Sanousi, a professor of language at Kuwait University, brought together a group of Muslim women in war-torn Kuwait, many of them premature widows, to write out their psychological and social suffering through third-person short stories. Before that, they had no voice. They found a release in expressing themes of hidden emotion and inner turmoil.

No matter where in the world you live, no matter how broken your life seems to be, the message comes through, loud and clear: Writing heals.

TECHNIQUES
TO GET YOU GOING

With Pen in Hand is almost a "best of techniques" book—a compilation of many methods I have either learned or invented over the years. For example, it adds an interesting dimension to what I call Branching (Chapter 12) and puts a new twist on

Interviewing the Critic (Chapter 9), both first introduced in *Writing on Both Sides of the Brain*.

In addition, here are some other techniques this book builds on:

Rapidwriting: Get It All Down

Every book I have written has the following premise: The kind of writing I advocate is not school writing, where perfect sentence A follows perfect sentence B, and you sit at a desk with a rigid-back chair, holding your hand at the correct angle. Rather, I recommend writing without restraint, capturing the "interior monologue," that is, writing without stopping to edit, correct, check for the right word. Get it all down first. Incorporate the static, the messages from your brain that say what you are writing is stupid and worthless. Do it anyway.

Twilight Writing: You Can Handle the Truth

Writing just as you are drifting off to sleep, or when you first begin to awake (notice, *not* get up) in the morning is a powerful way to access your inner knowing. I call it Twilight Writing, as in *The Twilight Zone.*

It is sometimes useful to pose a question the night before and let the subconscious work on it while you sleep (see Patti, Chapter 7). Then in the morning, before rising, before having a cup of coffee, going to the bathroom, or talking to anyone (all of which wakes up your left, analytical, brain)—Write. Pull the notebook into bed with you and move the pen automatically across the page in a somnambulistic state. You will be amazed at what comes out. In Twilight Writing, it is easier to tell the truth, because, as I like to put it, the Critic is still asleep. It is also an advantage for people who say they don't have the time to write.

It's okay to be sloppy and erratic in your penmanship. Keep moving forward—just don't try to cross your t's or dot your i's.

Resistance Has Meaning: Write Past Wanting to Stop

Writing is like climbing a hill on your bicycle. If you want to get to the top, don't get off the bike. Stay on the saddle. When you write, keep on writing, even if it gets hard. You can write about the difficulty, you can repeat what you just wrote, but don't get off the bike. Write about not wanting to write, how dumb it seems, how the words will not come, how they stick in your throat. Anything to get the pen moving across the page. If you feel resistant to writing, write about your resistance. Resistance has meaning.

Ask yourself, What is the obstacle to my healing, and am I ready to let go? Answer in writing until you get to something real.

Learn from Your Physical Self: Interview Your Body

Listen to your stomach, as Jennifer James likes to say.

Your body is trying to tell you something: your burning ears, the catch in your throat, the ache in your shoulders, all have a message for you.

If you can't bring yourself to write directly about your sorrow, concentrate on recording how you feel physically. The flared nostril, the itching eyes, the tight jaw: Describe it, and then ask, What is it telling me?

NOT GENERIC JOURNALING

For many, journal writing is a regular practice, and good for them. I want to be sure you understand, however, that what I am talking about here is not generic journaling. There are plenty of books already on the market about that. Personal writing as a way through grief embraces the non-writer, the occasional writer, the reluctant writer. *With Pen in Hand* offers a variety of ways to write to the reader who thinks that writing is linear, that writing is to be shared, that writing is to be polished. It provides a range of technique options, from interviewing the critic within, to writing a song or poem, from making lists to branching, from decorating a journal with more than the written word, to writing with the alternate hand.

The people in this book have been generous enough to share their experiences in order to help you through loss and grief in your own life. These people are not writers; many of them had never written before—or after.

After telling his or her individual story, each person interviewed answers in his or her own way this question: Why write? Why did writing make a difference?

Every answer is different.

And in each case, the chapter ends with the section Apply This. No matter what your own particular journey, you can learn from what others did, and adapt it to your own circumstances.

OTHERS HAVE WALKED THIS PATH

Jan is 55, going through a divorce after being married 23 years (see Chapter 2). Alone in her West Coast apartment, she writes,

> I wonder how many other people are feel-
> ing the way I do tonight?

Tim is 26, going on 27, without work, and he is feeling dis-
oriented (see Chapter 6). He sits on the opposite side of the
country, on the Great Lawn in Central Park,

> . . . looking at people around me and won-
> dering, are all these people as lost as I am or
> am I a special breed?

Perhaps the most important message of *With Pen in Hand:
The Healing Power of Writing* is this:

You are not alone.

Others have walked this path before you and they survived.

You will survive.

WITH PEN IN HAND

❧ CHAPTER 1 ❧

Why Writing Heals

My friend Parker is fond of a passage in the *Chronicles of Narnia*. The magician's nephew is on a winged horse in quest of the silver apple. Aslan tells him firmly that when he comes to the ice-mountain, he cannot fly over it; he has to go through it. That is the only way he will ever reach his true destination.

It is a truism of humanity. You cannot skirt the pain when your life is shattered by an event you never expected.

You must go through the mountain, not around it, not over it, and confront the snarling beasts and demons.

Fortunately, you have a tool to defend you and protect you, like a magic shield, a tool you were given in grade school. You don't even have to be good at it for it to work—and it is at your fingertips. Literally. Pick up your pen and write.

John, a reader from England, now living in the Canadian province of New Brunswick, sends me an E-mail telling about a horrific period in his life. His brother, then his father, died, and he almost lost his son through a bitter transcontinental custody battle. He thought he would go insane. He underlines for emphasis his salvation.

"The one action that has literally saved my life and my sanity, has been writing."

How is it that the simple act of putting pen to paper, of getting our thoughts out of our heads and onto the page can have this kind of power and curative effect?

WRITING PROVIDES GROUNDING

For one thing, making concrete marks out of abstract unarticulated thoughts provides grounding. It is a reality check.

When the foundation of life gives way, and you find yourself falling into a crater, writing puts earth back under your feet.

The act of consigning the hurricane inside your head to paper quiets the agitated spirit, shifts the brain waves, brings peace. It takes what can be toxic and decontaminates it. It makes it safe. Writing makes sense of confusion and gives voice to the wisdom within.

In *Put Your Heart on Paper*, I tell about 19-year-old Aaron Camp, who travels on a shoestring, sometimes with a one-way ticket. When he arrives at his destination, he has no place to go. Writing this fact down keeps him from panicking. For some reason, one stark example of his method has a hold on me. I use it verbatim when I am feeling lost:

> Here I am in San Francisco, I don't know
> where I am staying.

There. It's a fact. Now he can get his bearings and figure out what to do.

I call this Writing in Real-Time, as opposed to retrospective writing. (See Chapter 6, where Tim wrote about September 11th, recording the immediacy of the moment. Or Chapter 4, where Jenna noted what she was eating to get present.) Real-Time writing puts something solid under you when your world is shifting.

WRITING IS THERAPEUTIC

Often the best therapy is to voice your feelings and judgments to a sympathetic ear, to someone who won't turn on the ball-game or do the dishes, won't cradle the phone, multi-task, and tune you out. We usually have to pay for that kind of focused attention, but the secret is that by providing such a forum, the professional counselor leads you to find the answers inside yourself. And the best answers are the ones you already know, but don't know that you know.

You come to the aha! by spelling it out, by being given a platform to explore options. Writing does that. Writing brings you face-to-face with your own truth and reality. And truth and reality can set you free; otherwise, you are stuck.

The act of moving the pen across the page can be meditative, creating a calming state. Sometimes we don't even know what came out of our pen until we go back and read it later. And then we are surprised by the wisdom of our own words, and the insight.

My young friend Shane takes leave of a group of us talking together.

"Gotta go; I have an appointment with my therapist."

He grins and holds up his journal and heads off for a place where he can think and write in quiet.

WRITING IS HEALTHY

Researcher Dr. James Pennebaker of the University of Texas has spent the last 20 years examining, under laboratory conditions, the mind/body link between writing and health. More than simply a catharsis or venting, translating events into language can affect brain and immune functions. The subjects he tested had an increase in germ-fighting lymphocytes in their blood and lower stress levels. Pennebaker states that writing about emotional topics benefits health and also "has been found to reduce anxiety and depression, improve grades in college, and . . . aid people in securing new jobs."

Dr. Pennebaker tested a wide range of subjects, from "grade-school children and nursing home residents, arthritis sufferers, medical school students, maximum security prisoners, new mothers and rape victims." Writing about strong feelings improved the mental and bodily health of every category.

HAND VS. MACHINE:
TO WRITE OR TYPE

People often ask me, Is it okay to use the computer or a PDA (Personal Data Assistant)? Will it still work if I write electronically? Some people are more comfortable at the computer, others find it intrudes. Cassie (Chapter 8) likes the emotional distancing when she writes on her Mac. Some stalwart souls even use a typewriter, complete with inky ribbon and return carriage, with its satisfying little "bing!" at the end of each line. Whatever works for you is what is best. Whatever gets the words out of your head and onto the page is what is right.

If your usual mode is mechanical, however, I encourage you to try your hand at pen and paper. There is a different energy in it. Even choosing the writing tools can be a way of taking care of yourself—the pen that glides and has a heft you like, the notebook or journal with a picture or texture that invites you to relax. Many find comfort in the quiet and physicality of handwriting. The hand moving across the page can create a semi-trance. Some people have the ability to "zone out" while they are typing, but most find this "alpha state" easier to achieve while writing by hand. (If you do compose at the computer, turn off the monitor so you won't be tempted to tinker with the words as they appear before you. The idea is to write, not edit.)

GIVING OUT PERMISSION SLIPS

Judging from my mailbox, a lot of people are worried about doing it "right." There is no right, there is only do, as Yoda might say.

For several years now, I have been an "advice columnist," a kind of "Dear Abby," for a writing magazine. I answer questions about ways to journal.

People worry a lot about rules. One man, for example, wrote to ask, "Is it correct to use a Staedtler Mars Lumingraph 100 HB pencil?" A woman queried, "Is it okay to skip days in your journal?"

After a while, I came to realize that my specific answers to my readers did not matter. My job was to give out permission slips.

My stand is that there is no right or wrong way to write, and, I hope, through the anecdotes of others in *With Pen in Hand*, to give free access to all to use this powerful tool.

E-MAIL: THE COMMUNITY PIECE

My friend Rita used writing on the Internet to get her through a tough time. Her baby was sick with asthma, and her husband had been diagnosed with MS; in addition, Rita was battling a severe post-partum depression. The thought of writing by hand was overwhelming to her, but in the middle of the night, she found release through visiting an online MS chat room and through E-mail exchanges with a supportive person who was kind-hearted. She could write at any hour, agonizing at the keyboard over questions that had no answers. "Why me?" and "What part of Hell am I in now?"

Rita's writing solution is what Pennebaker calls "The Community Piece," because even though the people you are writing to are usually anonymous, there is a common caring and it is a relief to have that connection.

WHEN DO YOU
STOP FEELING THE PAIN?

Lisa (Chapter 3) cries when she talks about her baby who died 19 years ago. It's not that she is clinging to grief, but she will carry that child in her heart always.

The comedienne Linda Richman understands this. Devastated by her son's death in a car accident, and her mother's death a few days later, she wrote the book *I'd Rather Laugh*. A woman whose daughter died heard Richman speak and was surprised at how happy she seemed. After the presentation, the woman went up to Richman and asked, "When do you stop feeling the pain?"

"You don't," Richman answered.

"'You have to integrate the pain into your life,' I told her. 'It doesn't go away. It can't. It shouldn't. It's part of you. You had a beautiful child, and now you don't. That loss is part of you, just as your daughter was. These feelings are your feelings. What happened to you was hideous and horrible, and now you have to find a way to go on and even to rediscover laughter and joy.'"

HOLDING YOUR
HUMANITY IN OPEN HANDS

When your loss has been particularly devastating—and only you can judge that—there is no "closure."

"I hate that word, 'closure,'" says Jack Kennedy, the man who taught me so much about Ignatian Discernment (Chapter 5).

The television displays images of grieving parents at the site of a plane crash, family members walking through the ruins of a suicide bombing, the tanks withdrawing from the refugee camp. "And now let closure begin," intones the anchorman in a voiceover, as though there could ever be a termination of the emotions and pain in the face of such loss.

"Ignatius teaches how to hold the light and the darkness together," says Jack, citing the founder of the Jesuits, Ignatius of Loyola. "How do you hold a crying baby; how do you dress a wound? You take time and reverence. That's what I mean by 'holding.' It's okay to hold your grief—not hang on to it, but, in Dutch theologian Henri J. M. Nouwen's image, hold it with open hands. That's our humanity."

As Jack said that, it hit me like a thunderbolt. That is exactly what personal writing, in fact what this whole book, is all about. Not about closure, but about integration. About holding. With reverence. Whether a spiral drug store notebook, a leather-bound diary, or single sheets torn from a legal pad, the written page is a place to hold our humanity.

PLEASURE AND PAIN:
GATEWAY TO YOUR HUMANITY

Poet Mary Oliver put it this way: in order to be fully human, fully alive, "One or two things are all you need: / . . . some deep memory of pleasure, Some cutting / knowledge of pain."

Facing the sad emotions in your life tenderizes you to appreciate fully all the good that is there, too. Grief is not meant to shut you down, but to point to what is important.

Jack sums it up, "If you block your grief, you block your joy. They go together. The depth of joy can only be measured by your willingness to go to your depth of sadness. What you discover is how deep you are."

EMILY'S PENCIL CASE:
A MANTRA FOR MY LIFE

I am supposed to be exactly where I am.

I know that because my daughter Emily told me so, and even hand-painted it on my favorite, carry-it-with-me-every-day-of-my-life canvas pencil case. Against a backdrop of deep purple, Emily scrolled my name in yellow above the zipper, with a mountain range in wild strokes of blues and greens pictured underneath. At the highest peak, she drew a woman in exaltation, (presumably me) arms flung wide, foot lifted in a high kick, with a full sun behind her. Below the dancing figure it reads,

I am supposed to be exactly where I am.

Sometimes when I am traveling, I use the pouch as a little purse, so I had it with me when I got lost in the cobblestone alleys of Athens. I couldn't find my way back to Dhionissiou Areopayitou, the main boulevard. The narrow, winding stepped streets up the slopes of the Acropolis, the stark white houses of the Plaka all looked the same; nothing looked familiar. I started to panic. Then I looked down at the pencil case in my hand with its comforting inscription. I took it literally. This is where I am supposed to be; don't be afraid. And soon I found my way.

Many times now I go back to that motto and it reminds me that I am not lost, or dumb, or anything less than what I am meant to be—physically, geographically, emotionally, financially, spiritually. Even stuck in traffic: I am supposed to be exactly where I am.

Writing is like my painted pencil case from Emily—writing reminds you that it is okay to be you, whatever that means. Accept what is. "It's okay to be sad," says Pinkly, a survivor of domestic violence (Chapter 14). Mike (Chapter 13), who lived through Vietnam, echoes her. How you do things is not how somebody else does things. Writing lets you heal at your own stride. Writing will not hurry you along or get impatient with you.

You are supposed to be exactly where you are.

STAY IN THE MIDST

Taking time is counter culture. We want an instant answer.

Jack presents an alternative view.

"You need to stay until you know where you are. If you try to move beyond where you are at, you get to come back to where you are at anyway. If you stay long enough, it will shift and lead you to the next organic place of itself."

That is exactly the role of writing. Writing supports you in staying in the midst of it until it shifts.

The world is impatient. It tells you, You should be over that by now. The page does not judge how long it takes you. The page can hold your sorrow and will not rush you on.

Honor your inner life and trust the process.

When you have a mind-boggling loss in your life, or have lived through war, sexual abuse, domestic violence, or other trauma, you need to heal on your own time frame. Nobody but you can say how long that takes.

And that is where writing comes in. Writing allows you to integrate, at your own pace.

LABOR LEADS TO BIRTH

Those of you who have given birth, or been present at the scene, know that the toughest part of labor is the period right before delivery. That's when the mother wants to quit—as if it were possible!—and the labor coach is all smiles. He has read the books and taken the classes, and he knows the signs: The baby is almost here. The tougher it gets, the closer the birth.

Do you know what this duration is called?

Transition.

Isn't that apt?

Transition is a bridge; it is going somewhere. Right after the most strenuous stretch, something glorious is waiting. Something worth working for, worth hanging in there and pushing for when you don't feel like pushing. After the pain comes new life.

Think of your writing as an infinitely patient and caring labor coach. You are in transition. You can't fly over it, you have to go through it. There will always be a way through. Remember to breathe.

How does writing help heal? Come see.

CHAPTER 2

Divorce Was Like a Death

The Death of the Dream

Waiters and waitresses call them "campers"—those who sit for hours in a restaurant, nursing the after-meal coffee or Coke. I was so engrossed in Jan's tale, so engaged by her natural humor, the intensity and sincerity of her aquamarine eyes, that I didn't notice how many times the server at Mitzel's American Kitchen presented the check to me.

We had met at this very restaurant, off the interstate, midway between our two houses, over five years ago, when Jan told me the story of her baby Justine dying, for the book I was writing then, *Put Your Heart on Paper*. Now she had a different loss to discuss, and once again, writing has helped in her healing.

"Divorce is like a death," she said. "The death of the dream."

It surprised me to hear her say that, since she was the one who chose to leave, and almost instantly, had a boyfriend interested in her. I did not expect her to be sad.

Jan and Gladwin were married 23 years.

She admits it: As difficult as the marriage was, it was still devastating to get divorced.

THE IMPETUS TO LEAVE

Jan met Michael at a party.

"He was a lot of fun; he was very attentive. I needed attention; he gave it to me. I had been ignored for so long. I was like a starving person.

"He gave me a kick in the butt—the courage to make a decision that I had been wanting to make for years. I thought, There are men out there in the world who will talk to me; and there are people who care about me. Maybe I don't have to be stuck in this dead marriage for the rest of my life."

That's when she started looking for an apartment.

And that was when she began writing about her situation on big white pads of lined legal paper, with sheets that tore off at the top.

> As the children grew more independent, I felt the emptiness in my heart, realizing I wasn't going to be able to endure it too much longer. I began to entertain the idea of finding the courage to leave Gladwin. Meeting Mike propelled me onward—onward to a place I had no idea could be both so freeing and so lonely.

LONELY HEART,
LONELY PLACE TO LIVE

At first, she was glad and excited.

"The day I signed the lease for the apartment, I was dancing. I'm free! I'm finally free. I thought, I have my own apartment; I am out of there; at last I am happy. I don't have to deal with all the things that were bothering me."

She says now she was in shock, not thinking correctly.

"I had no idea, no consideration of the fact that one day I might feel pain."

Then it was like novocaine subsiding and exposing the real feeling beneath.

"The happiness wore off, the 'I'm free!' wore off. And then I got very sad. Then the pain hit. It was all but unbearable."

It came on fast and fierce, almost in one day.

"All of a sudden, I started sobbing. What have I done?

"The short time of happiness from getting to leave went bye-bye, and then I was awake."

> This pain of being alone won't let go. I was alone in my twenty-three year marriage, but this is a different kind of alone. In those many years of being alone with Gladwin, I had my babies and my friends. I was busy for so long I didn't have time to face the reality of a desolate marriage. My life was still fulfilling and it seemed to balance out.
>
> Yet the changes I'm experiencing are far more difficult than I ever could have

anticipated. The grieving has begun—for the dream that never happened. The dream of happy marriage and family.

She did not like being alone in her tiny new apartment.

I thought I would love having my space, and now sometimes I loathe it. Sometimes, especially on sunny summer evenings, I just drive in my car listening to CDs rather than going "home." I feel as if I don't have a home anymore. Like I don't belong anywhere.

I have no yard, no flowers, no garden, no animals, few trees, no patio. Just some cement stairs leading to a cement sidewalk, leading to blacktop where I get into my car and leave.

Sometimes she felt so lost, it was like being in the middle of a prairie full of nothing but tumbleweed.

This apartment is so lonely. That must be why it is called an APART ment. I feel apart from everything—isolated and many miles away from how I used to be. It's all part of this process called divorce. It has left me feeling vulnerable and weak. I hate this feeling. I feel like I've lost my identity—as a wife and mother. When you are in that role for so many years you become enmeshed with it. It is a 24-hour-a-day, 365-day-a-year job and now that it's gone, I feel lost. I did not have a CLUE that it would be like this. I have to rediscover who I am inside and separate that from the role I've played for so long. And that will take time—longer than I think.

My heart is so sad. My life is undone. So many broken dreams. I feel this deep gnawing pain in the center of my being, like being kicked in the gut a thousand times.

WHY SHE LEFT

When Gladwin and Jan were together, they lived with financial pandemonium. Gladwin is an independent contractor. It was either feast or famine.

The repetitive scene was almost comic, but at the time, it did not seem very funny.

"When he came home at night, I followed him down the hall, trying to find out if he had any money. He went to the bedroom, and locked the door. That's what he did, locked himself in a room. Go in a door, shut it on me; go out a door, and shut it; go to the truck, and shut the door—anything to avoid confrontation, communication of any kind."

One of the main reasons Jan left was the never knowing.

"I would call them bad surprises: a sign on the house that there was going to be a sheriff's sale; a notice in the mail that the insurance lapsed. From the public utility, a cut-off notice. The telephone being turned off. Or I would come out and my car had been towed away, repossessed. Household goods at the pawnshop."

Jan believes that Gladwin means well, that deep down, he wants to improve.

"But I never saw evidence of it. It's as if he has a brain warp in the area of finances.

"Now I grieve for my kids, and myself, because my dream of the perfect marriage, or at least a good marriage, didn't happen. I was the kind of person who did not think divorce was an option. I swore, other than physical abuse, I would stay committed, no matter what."

> Gladwin is a man with many wonderful qualities, but those qualities couldn't outweigh the years of dealing with his business, and the constant chaos it caused. I would never have left if I thought there was even a tiny bit of hope. So now I'm starting at square one. Starting over—like I'm 18 again, and trying to decide what to be when I grow up.

ONE INCH OF PAPERWORK

The forms to fill out, the documents to gather, the information to verify, was grueling. And shifting through it was a heartache.

> I have a stack of paperwork an inch thick to tackle for the "dissolution" of our marriage. What a word, dissolve—dissolving our family, a way of life. Doing that paperwork is an emotional drain. It's all so sad. It's hard to say good-bye, even to what was a rough marriage.

Jan realizes that she probably has a lot of company going through the stages of grief, but that doesn't make it any easier.

> I wonder how many other people are feeling the way I do tonight? Probably millions. Life is definitely a road with countless hills, valleys, curves, barriers, and dead ends. It's a damn hard journey a lot of the time. I have survived so far, sometimes surmounting nearly impossible challenges. Of course I can see that looking back. Today, though, I'm having trouble even drawing on the previous victories I've had. I'm blank today—like someone wiped out the slate that stored all my strength. And damn it I need that today. Maybe tomorrow something good will happen. I need something to inspire me. Please God—send me some inspiration. If you don't—I swear I'll die. And that wasn't really in my plans yet.

THINKING BACK
TO THE HAPPY TIMES

Jan starts to cry softly as she talks about being at the airport recently and seeing a dad come up to the fence with his two little boys. He had stopped so they could watch the planes take off.

"It caused me to recall, with tears ready to pour out, those days so many years ago when Gladwin and I would take the children to do things like that: watch airplanes, or boats, or trains, or animals. We all had so much fun. It was the happiest time of my life."

> I saw a dad at Eagle Hardware, holding his little boy's hand as they walked through the aisle of nuts and bolts and screws. I almost lost it. It reminded me of Gladwin and our son Joel. One thing: he was (is) a patient, kind, loving, and attentive dad. He always loved his kids.

She misses those times, and to her surprise, even longs for the clamor and confusion that used to drive her crazy.

> It is so quiet. I miss having people around making noise, talking, eating, joking, bitching, laughing, loving, needing, making messes —all that a family is composed of. I am going through withdrawal.
>
> Nothing is familiar anymore. Familiar, of course, comes from the word family. My family has disintegrated. I am starting over. I wanted to do this. But after so many years of being part of a family (in fact, the hub of a family), I wasn't prepared for the multitude of things that disintegrate. And the huge effect it has on me.

Holidays were tough, especially Christmas.
"We have cathedral ceilings, sixteen feet high, so we always had a tall beautiful noble fir. We used a ladder to decorate it."

Christmas is in three weeks. It will be so different for all of us this year. What about the beautiful Christmas tree we always had? Will Gladwin put it up and decorate it? I don't know. I just wish this season were over. I hate it.

A holiday compounds everything because it's a family time, and my family has been broken.

At times like these, she was unmerciful in her judgment of herself.

I have ruined the family. It's all my doing. I couldn't stay anymore. Couldn't I have stayed—hung in there, to keep my family intact? But I was dying on the vine. So many obstacles over the years had made me empty, unable to take one more step to stay in the 20+ years of such craziness. Yet, I remember how it once was. The most important thing to do for your kids is to love each other, and be good role models. And I failed in the marriage department.

And she thinks about the man who was her husband and what he must be going through.

I cry for Gladwin because though we were not a good combination for marriage I still love him as a person and I hurt for him. I

know his heart is empty and broken. And I
can't do anything about it.

THE EMPTY
FEELING OF THE HOUSE

After Jan left, she would go back to the house to straighten up,
feed the animals, and do the laundry. She says the house was
like a dead body.

"The spirit had gone out of the house. When the mother is
not there, something leaves; the house was like a dead house.
When we were a family there, there was a oneness, the family
unit; now the circle of energy had been broken.

"After I moved out it was awful."

> I went out to what was once my beautiful
> garden to pick some flowers for the house.
> Then I picked some raspberries among the
> two-ft.-high weeds. It was so sad. The whole
> dream life has crashed into bits and pieces.
> Even the animals seemed lost and lonely.

"The dog would go nuts, jump all over me, and follow me
and lick me. She was a mama's girl dog; I was her mom. I would
say to myself, You left your dog. You are a bad dog mother."

> The dogs and cats seem confused that I don't
> live there anymore. Today when I went to
> go, I petted Pepper. I can tell she misses
> me. She may be just a dog, but she's my dog,

and she thinks I'm her "mother." And her "mother" abandoned her.

And the horse would stare at her and whinny.

Ziggy, my horse, comes immediately to nicker and nuzzle me with his nose. He used to be so hard to catch. Now he loves to rub his cheek against my face and wants to ride.

There are so many losses involved in divorce. I have to grieve and get past each one of them. Since I wanted to leave, I didn't know I would not be immune to the grieving. I was so happy to leave, how could I know I would still be so sad about what was left behind? I cry a lot. My emotions are raw.

As sad as the house seemed, it was wrenching when it came time to sell it.

I found out Wednesday that the house had been sold. Another piece of a dream that's broken. My children won't have the home they grew up in to come home to. When I think of the memories, good and bad, it makes me sob. I remember when we were building it—the fun and the anxiety all part of the picture, the picture of my life that has been ripped apart. It is going to be difficult if not impossible to drive up Dubuque

Road. To see someone else parked in the driveway will be too hard for me.

LIKE JUSTINE'S
DEATH IN SO MANY WAYS

The anguish Jan was enduring felt familiar. She had been there before.

> It's December again—my least favorite month of the year. I can't believe it's been nine years since Justine died. The horrible searing pain of those first months and years is gone. I would not want to relive that time for anything. Now years later, I'm in another sad situation. Our divorce will be final on December 20th. And the pain is very much like pain of losing my Justine. Broken dreams. Both the baby and the marriage.

Jan says that there is a reason that she knows divorce is the same as death.

"After Justine died, a wave of sadness would come over me without warning; I would hear a song and start crying, gut-crying. We're talking a wailing cry, not just a surface cry, coming from your heart, from the deepest part of you."

She has had that same thing happen since the divorce.

"I am driving along or out shopping, and there is a trigger. I am at Dunn Lumber, and my eye falls on a brochure with a picture of windows exactly like those in my old house, down to the paint, the exact same color that I had painted my house. I start sobbing; I have to go outside.

"A picture of a window made me sad out of nowhere."

> I sit here, frozen, afraid to venture out. I can't believe it's me, Jan, feeling so small and inadequate. I don't ever remember feeling like this since Justine died. Only now, I'm on my own. I hurt so much for my family. I never wanted it to be like this. I don't think anyone does.
>
> I put so much time and energy into something that didn't work. For nothing? It reminds me of being pregnant with Justine just to have her die.

"I guess there was a death—my life as I knew it, or my life as I wished it had been—has died."

MICHAEL NOT FAMILY:
HOW COULD HE KNOW?

Michael could not make the sadness go away. She did not expect him to.

> Michael has been a great help and a diversion from the pain—yet he certainly isn't the answer to it all—he's just a man, and no human being can fill the void of a life left behind.

"I am lonely even though I have a boyfriend. He is not my kids' father; he is not my family. He wasn't my husband of 23 years; he wasn't my animals' father who had been with me through all of the stuff we had gone through, all the memories, good and bad.

"He is not what would make my fragmented family be whole. He can't fix it. Just as someone else's baby can't ever replace mine."

Jan's oldest daughter, Julianna, recently turned 21.

"I couldn't talk to Michael about how I felt; it wouldn't mean anything to him. Gladwin was the one who was there when she was born and saw her first smile."

Jan just generally hated the newness of dating.

> Dating feels so strange to me now after so many years of being married. When I was single, I got so sick of the whole dating scene. And now I remember why. I love the joy that it brings; yet there is a risk in sharing your heart with another person so intimately. What would happen should we ever part ways? And why doesn't he call?

Sitting by the phone waiting for it to ring took Jan back thirty years or more, and made her feel like a flighty teenager.

> God, how I hated waiting for a guy to call. Stuck. Waiting for calls that sometimes came and sometimes didn't. It used to make me crazy—and here I am doing it again.

But what else do I have to do tonight?
My little tiny apartment is clean. I am not
married anymore, not the mother of little
ones who need me.

"I get insecure when he doesn't call. My mind wanders and
starts thinking maybe he's backing off."

Maybe he is trying to dump me, and I am
too dense to see it.

"Whereas when you're married, even if it is not perfect, you
have a more stable feeling."
Jan was afraid to tell Michael how much she needed him.

I care deeply for him, but he doesn't have a
clue how lonely I am and I guess I don't
want him to know. It's a game. I have to act
like I'm fine. And I'm not. He couldn't
handle me needing him too much.

Jan had been alone in her marriage years on end. And now
she wanted to be with someone.

A lot. Not just part time. I don't want to be
low on his list of things to do; I want to
be close to the top.
Michael has been single for a long time.
He's accustomed to being alone. How
could he understand what it's like for me?

BEING IN BOOT CAMP

Jan is sure that one day she will be able to see the good in all this.

> I'll live in the reality of a new life. Fear will dissipate, security will return, my former confidence will emerge with amazing new strength. If I can just get through "these days," that "one day" will come.

She has an analogy that helps her to understand the growth, the formidable task, and the fact that this period is not permanent, but something she will move on from.

"This time of loss and grief is like being in boot camp—so hard, yet bringing with it a discipline learned no other way than through being pushed beyond your limits."

> I feel like giving up sometimes (like at least ten times a day) but I can't. So I have to imagine that I'm in boot camp and it's tough—but I will get through, and when I do, I'll be tougher and stronger, and more able to face challenges in life.

And she acknowledges the reality that her marriage was not healthy, for either of them.

"My husband and I brought out the worst in each other. Both of our true identities were dormant for all those years."

Now the real Jan is coming alive.

"The person locked inside of me for so long has finally started to live the way I believe I was meant to."

> It is all part of a difficult transition I have to walk through one day at a time. I'll survive, and even thrive when I'm down the road a little further, but I still cry now. I know I will come out of this with renewed strength and character (though I hate the process of building character!).

Jan is working toward independence. She is setting up an espresso stand at a "Park and Ride" municipal bus station. Her partner has good business sense; Jan has a knack with coffee and with customers.

"Between his head and my people strengths, we will make the business go. In this coffee-loving state that we live in, it will be successful."

And meantime, she has a peace and a freedom.

"Even though I may not have much money, I know what I do have. I know how much I earn, and how much I owe. I know what my budget is.

"I am not depending on somebody's word that there is money coming in. There are no surprises. Finances are now in my charge, rather than being out of control. This is a good thing."

Jan has a goal for another comfort that would mean a lot to her.

"I would like to see a day come when I can call Gladwin as a friend and say, How're you doing? The kids are up to this or that. That is a freedom I am working toward."

WHY WRITE?

Some people write, then burn what they wrote. Jan sometimes hides her journals, but she could not destroy them.

"Those pages are precious to me. I don't write them to throw away. Even though it sometimes makes me cry to reread what I wrote."

Why would you want to write something that would make you cry? Something you would have to hide?

"Writing is my release. Stress causes tension, and tension causes headaches, back pain and shoulder aches. You have to have a valve to let off the steam. You will find a discharge one way or the other, why not do it with writing, because it's safer?

"Fear causes more tension; it's a cycle. Writing turns the light on; the anxiety is gone."

When Jan's baby died, she couldn't sleep, so she would get up in the middle of the night and write.

"I still do that. Writing is like a tranquilizer."

> Today the pain is almost intolerable. The circuits in my brain, or heart, are blowing. They're all mixed up, not on the right pathways as they should be.
>
> Writing helps a lot—I feel a bit more sane already.

Also, Jan says, a journal becomes a barometer, a way to compare where she was with where she is now.

"I found my old journal from nine years ago, when the baby died, and read the first five or six pages of it. That's why I would never throw anything away. Looking back, it was good to see I wasn't there anymore, in that horrible place of grief that I thought I would never get out of.

"I actually could read it. It made me cry a little, because of the emotion involved; but the pain, the searing agonizing pain that wouldn't go away that I wrote about isn't there anymore.

"There were days when I wrote, 'I don't see how my heart keeps beating.' I used to pray, Please God, heal this broken heart—and I never believed it would happen. It did. I no longer suffer from that particular grief. My heart has been restored."

Jan says reading that old journal was a reminder.

"I will get through this present sadness, because I got through the other grief. I thought I was going to die, but I didn't."

Remarkably, Jan can now see the good that came forth out of the sorrow of her baby's death, the depth of compassion that she would not have any other way.

"There is something precious that comes out of grief, but it is not going to show its face for a long time. When it does, you will see that what you sow in tears, you will reap in joy."

Jan is pragmatic about writing, even when she does not feel like doing it.

> I don't want to work out, but I need to do
> that too.

"Even though I hate going to the gym, I'm always glad I went. I don't know why that is. I don't know why getting on the treadmill releases endorphins in the brain, but it does."

> When I am in the middle of working out at
> the club, it's hard, hot, sweaty, and my mus-
> cles burn. But when I leave, I feel so good.

And—even better—after one year of faith-
fully working out, I can see some awesome
results.

When you're in the midst of the fire and
heat—well, that's not when you see the
strength coming. It's when you feel your
weakest, that you're getting the strongest.

Jan is emphatic, like a mother telling you to eat your vegeta-
bles and drink your milk.

"Writing and exercise: you don't have to know why they
work. They are means to an end. Just do it."

After awhile, you will see some awesome results.

APPLY THIS

In *Deor's Lament,* the medieval minstrel catalogues all the
calamities that have befallen the kingdom over the years as an
exhortation not to lose heart in the present troubles. Each verse
ends with the refrain, "That evil ended, so also may this."

Use your past writing as a benchmark of your progress.

Looking back, you will see how far you have come.

"That evil ended, so also may this."

Writing is part of the process that gets you to the other side.
You may not feel like writing. Do it anyway.

CHAPTER 3

A Lullaby for
a Baby Who Died

Turning Sadness into Song

Dale and I go way back. We were members of the National Speakers Association together. In the 1980s he showed me the draft of a book he wrote for little children, *Over Is Not Up*, about a little girl named Bitsie, who doesn't want to get up in the morning. I thought it was terrific, and encouraged him to publish it. Years later, he and his daughter Lisa co-authored *The Secrets of Rebel Cave*, a young adult novel about the Civil War and World War II, and I was delighted to be their editor. I fell in love with the characters, Jackie, Dulcie, Hattie, and I fell in love with Dale and Lisa. It was a joy to work with them.

It was then that Dale told me something I didn't know. *Over Is Not Up* was dedicated to his granddaughter, Lisa's child, who died after open-heart surgery. Lisa herself had written a lullaby for this baby. Dale marvels at this combination of tributes.

"*Over Is Not Up* is a beautiful book that thousands of boys and girls love. In the front, it says, 'To the memory of Elizabeth Anne (Betsie). Our Itsie Bitsie Betsie is UP.' I told Lisa that not many wee infants have inspired both an award-winning book and a published and recorded song. So the 'tiny babe in the tiny grave tucked away in a quiet place' has been far better immortalized than she would have been with a splendid marble or granite marker."

One winter morning on what turned out to be her birthday, I called Lisa in Wisconsin to talk to her about her baby and her song. It has been 19 years since her baby died, yet the details she shared with me are as fresh as today. A number of times in our long conversation, I had to put the phone down, and take a deep breath. There were times when we were both crying—and then laughing at ourselves, almost in disbelief. How could we be touched all these years later by a little life that lasted seven days?

NOTHING PREPARES YOU

In a clear strong alto voice, Lisa begins our conversation by singing the opening verse of her ballad to her baby.

> *There's a tiny babe in a tiny grave*
> *Tucked away in a quiet place.*
> *And a mother's heart nearly broke apart*
> *When they laid her child away.*
> *It was long ago, ten years or so,*

But the pain is still inside.
If you listen near you can almost hear
What the grieving mother cried.

It may seem stark to use the word "grave," but death is stark, Lisa says.

"Death is raw, death is cold earth tossed to the side. That's what death is. Nothing in my life prepared me for how I felt when my baby died."

THE BABY'S BIRTH AND HEART

Lisa and her husband, Rick, were living in San Antonio when she found out she was expecting their third child.

"Right from the start, it felt like a gift to be pregnant again, because it wasn't something we thought would happen. We waited in anticipation and eagerness."

The baby was born on February 16, six weeks early, at Memphis Hospital. She weighed 4 pounds, 15 ounces. Lisa is an Army-trained nurse, so she knew right away something was wrong. The baby was immediately rushed from the delivery room into the Neonatal Intensive Care Unit, where they did a sonogram of her heart. There appeared to be some major heart defects. She was transferred to the University of Texas Health Center in San Antonio Hospital to have an ecocardiogram done.

"They brought her back after the eco and told us she had transposition of the great vessel. That meant that the oxygen-carrying vessels that come out of the left side of her heart turned right around and went back into the same side."

The doctors did a balloon systostemy to open up a hole to give the baby more oxygen in her blood. Her chances were not good, but the physicians said if they could keep the baby alive until she was a year old, they could do corrective surgery. Because the baby's heart was so small, it would be dangerous to do it sooner.

"We are talking about a heart the size of a walnut, little tiny vessels like spaghetti, or smaller—vermicelli vessels."

Lisa spent her days at the hospital with the baby, and her nights at home with Tracy, her three-year-old, and Rickie, her one-year-old. Then back to the hospital she'd go, every morning.

They named the baby Elizabeth Anne with an "e" on the end of Anne.

Lisa chuckles, remembering how they shortened that immediately.

"She was so little that it seemed like that was just too big a name. So we called her Betsie almost from the moment she was born."

Even though she was very sick, Betsie was soft and new and pure.

"She was a sweet baby girl, a little Xerox copy of my older two, except that her hair had a touch of red."

When Betsie was seven days old, she had congestive heart failure. The doctors said, We have to do the surgery now.

"Mom and Dad drove down from Kentucky that morning, so they were able to see her and touch her and pray over her. Right before they took her in, Daddy held her. He is a big man. She had lost eight ounces and now weighed only four and a half pounds. She was dwarfed in his hand."

Dale picked her up, and he said, "Oh, Lisa. It's not like holding a baby. It's like holding a warm feeling."

The finality of the next sentence is hard, even now, for Lisa to say. She takes a gulp of air to brace herself.

"She had a wonderful surgical team, but she did not survive the surgery."

Here Lisa inhales again deeply, and slowly lets it out, as yet once again, the horror of those words sink in. There is a long pause, and then, in a low voice, she sums up the rest of her life.

"And so began my journey."

GRIEF — THE JOURNEY

"For me, emotionally, they are horribly, horribly, horribly dark months. I can't say horribly enough times or underline it enough."

Betsie died on Wednesday; she was buried on Thursday. The following Tuesday, Lisa went back to work.

"I couldn't think, it was like my brain was no longer capable of putting thoughts together. I found myself falling into periods where I had no awareness of time passing. I had two babies on the floor; I couldn't just space out and not be there. So I went back to work because I felt like I was losing my mind. Going to work would force me to my senses."

Lisa stutters when she describes the physical reaction.

"It, it was the most bizarre thing. My arms ached; my arms literally ached, and I felt like I was choking all the time. I thought I was insane."

Lisa had not brought either of the other children to the hospital. In hindsight, she wishes she had, even though they were just babies themselves.

"Tracy in particular did not understand why we did not bring this baby home. We had talked about the baby. She was going to 'help Mommy take care of the baby.' 'When our baby comes, we'll do this' . . . 'When our baby comes, we'll do that,' and when our baby came, she never came home."

For months after Betsie died, when they went to visit friends and spend the evening with them, Tracy wanted to go out and sleep in their car when it got to be about eight o'clock. It took Lisa a while to figure out what she was doing.

She was making sure that she got taken home.

"Isn't that something? You just don't realize the profound effect the loss of a child can have on anyone, much less your three-year-old."

Holidays were especially hard. Easter was the first major holiday after Betsie died.

"I couldn't do Easter. I couldn't make two baskets; I needed to make three baskets. And I couldn't make three baskets, because that would have meant I was deranged. My sister-in-law made Easter baskets for each of my kids.

"I let Rickie and Tracy have their Easter egg hunt, and I enjoyed it with them but I could not do it myself.

"I saw absolutely no peace in my future, no beauty, no laughter, no song. Nothing positive in my future right at that moment."

THE THINGS THAT PEOPLE SAY

Probably because they are at a loss for words, people often express sentiments meant to console a bereaved parent that do anything but. Some offered platitudes such as "You should be thankful for the children you have."

Lisa's response to that one was immediate.

"I know I have other children, and I am thankful. But children are not lightbulbs. They don't burn out and you say, Oh well, I've got two more on the shelf."

Then there were those who suggested piously that it must have been the Lord's will.

"That one just frosted me.

"I have huge faith. And one of the things I have faith in is that God is a loving God. I don't believe he sits up in heaven and says, Here's a family that have been going along for awhile doing pretty well, let's give them a sick baby."

Lisa believes that God allows certain things to happen, and when he does, "we have a responsibility to walk by faith through the valley and to hold on to his hand, and not try to do it by ourselves.

"But I don't believe that God throws lightning bolts through a baby's heart. God does not will a child to die."

People mean well. They think that since it made Lisa sad to talk about the baby, it would be better not to ask. Lisa is emphatic in decrying how misguided that reasoning is.

"So many people acted like she never was, like I'd never had that pregnancy at all. And that hurt so badly. It caused deep pain when people acted like it never happened. I know now with the distance of time that people don't mean to be cruel. Their intention is to be kind, but if you never ask me, then by not validating her death, you invalidate her life.

"She was a *real* person. She had a name. She had arms and legs and fingers and toes, and big brown eyes and strawberry blond hair and the family scowl. She could draw those little eyebrows down and wrinkle up her forehead just like my other two children. She was *real*. She was a person, with a soul. And I'm one of the few people who knew her."

Lisa had a great need to talk about her baby. She uses a comparison that she says shocks people because they do not understand.

"I realize it sounds disgusting, but particularly in the first year after her death, the need for me to talk about her was like the need to vomit. I couldn't stop. It was physically impossible for me *not* to express myself about this baby and about her death, and about her life, and about the unfairness of it all."

Lisa felt ripped off. She had had an ultrasound. She knew it was a high-risk pregnancy because of an Rh factor, but they were not prepared for a heart defect.

"It came out of *no*where and blindsided me. Somehow in your mind you know that you will lose your grandparents, and probably your parents, but you don't expect to lose your children."

It was like somebody cheated in the middle of the game.

"They pulled an ace out of their sleeve, and said, mockingly, You lose!"

It was because of that profound sense of being *robbed* that Lisa had to talk about her baby.

"If I didn't, I was afraid she would disappear. Somebody had to talk about her, and I was her mom. So that became my job."

Lisa also found herself holding on tightly to anything that was connected, even in a loose way, with Betsie.

"It's funny the things that we *cling* to. My sister-in-law's mother gave me an African violet while the baby was in the hospital, so I had it at the same time I had her. And I nursed that little potted plant, and took care of it, and when that African violet died, I felt like I'd lost Betsie all over again. Because it was a link, a link to her."

A POEM ABOUT A CRADLE

Another link was the baby's cradle, complete with little soft blankets. It was all made up, still waiting for the baby who would never come home. It stayed in Rick and Lisa's bedroom for months; she could not bring herself to store it in the attic, even when Rick asked, Isn't it time to put the cradle away?

Richard himself had surprised Lisa with the cradle at Christmas. They hadn't had a cradle for the older two. He joined the pieces of unvarnished wood together, sanded it and shellacked it. That wooden bed with rockers, meant to lull the newborn babe to sleep, was now a symbol of their emptiness and loss. In Lisa's mind, it would always be unfinished, because it never got to hold her baby.

In the first attempt that she can pinpoint of putting her pain on paper, Lisa wrote a poem called "The Unfinished Cradle."

"I had used writing as a cathartic exercise before in my life; this was certainly the biggest test."

In the poem she describes how "Daddy joined the newcut wood" and put the cradle under the tree, how she herself lovingly touched the grain with longing, anticipating the baby who would soon rest there. But it was not to be.

You came to us one night so fast
But your life was not to last.
Fate spit out her cruelest joke,
Your heart stopped, my heart broke.

"It took me a long time to bring myself to write that poem. Seeing it spelled out was harsh."

SUPPORTED BY
COMPASSIONATE FRIENDS

Lisa did not know where to turn in her despair. She joined a bereaved parents support group called Compassionate Friends.

"Compassionate Friends is one of the things that saved me from absolute oblivion. Knowing that I wasn't alone, that the pain that I was feeling was not insanity but normal grief was incredibly, incredibly important. Maybe I am not so crazy after all; if these parents felt deranged sometimes, I guess it's normal that I feel that way, too."

Lisa was touched by the range of other families who were there.

"There was one mother whose son died in Vietnam, and she was still coming to meetings. There were elderly people whose grown children had died in car accidents; there were SIDS [sudden infant death syndrome] parents; there were parents whose children had had horrible diseases, and there was one set of parents whose child had had a double liver transplant and had died after the second one failed. It was impossibly moving to be with these other parents and see their pain, and their healing, to know that they had *survived*."

One mother at a meeting had on nail polish; another was wearing makeup. These may seem like ordinary, taken-for-granted things, but instead they became a beacon that life might one day return to some kind of normalcy.

"I did not think I was going to survive; I truly did not believe I could live. But when I saw them, I knew I could and would."

Richard came too, reluctantly.

It was at a Compassionate Friends meeting that one of the fathers said, "I get so angry when people say, 'How is your wife doing?' like the baby wasn't mine, too."

That remark startled Lisa awake.

"Hearing that brought me to an awareness that I had not been facing: this was not just my pain. I knew that Rick was grieving, but his grief was so silent that it didn't seem like it hurt him as badly as it hurt me. On an intellectual level, I knew that was not true, but he wasn't the one struggling to get out of bed in the morning, or if he was, he wasn't letting me know."

Her voice chokes up as she continues.

"It was difficult for me to accept that it wasn't just my pain. It was an important thing for me to hear. And it was important for Rick to hear that he wasn't the only one."

And that's when Lisa realized it was time to put the cradle away.

"After hearing that father at the meeting share, it dawned on me that as much comfort as having that cradle was giving me, it was giving him an equal amount of pain. So I put the cradle away. It was time. I was able to look past my own pain, and get a glimpse of his. I took the cradle down, and took it apart, and put it away."

SO FEW THINGS

It was many years later before she was able to give the cradle to someone else.

"Many, many years later. Because we had so few things that were hers. A couple of preemie sleepers and some little tiny stuffed animals that I had bought at the hospital gift shop and put in her isolette, and that was it. Her birth certificate and her death certificate. Condolence cards. There is not a lot to prove that this baby was. I have a small box inside my Hopechest that

I call the Betsie Box. It has one of her sleepers in it and her little animals, sympathy cards. . . "

Her voice cracks, she starts to cry.

"That's my Betsie Box."

LOVE WITHOUT LIFE

For several years, Lisa stayed involved with the Alamo chapter of Compassionate Friends. She was the one they called when there were new baby deaths, to make the first contact with the stricken parents.

When the chapter was contacted by a group looking for a keynote speaker, they knew Lisa was the ideal choice.

"The conference was called 'Love Without Life,' a wonderfully articulate name. That's exactly what it is. You have all this love for this being that is no more."

The audience was composed of doctors, nurses, and caregivers from area hospitals. The conference was for prenatal and perinatal loss miscarriages, stillbirths, specifically early loss.

Lisa had never been asked to give a speech before. What would she say? When she finally sat down to write, the words poured out of her like lava, and touched again a tender spot.

She sobbed over the pages as she wrote. When she finished, she had fourteen single-spaced, typed pages. She pared it down to two.

"I wanted to tell everything. Every moment of her life, every breath she took, every procedure that she had: everything. Then logic kicked in. 'You are writing a speech to be given to other people. Okay, let's hit the highlights.'"

Lisa rehearsed her remarks, and talked it through with her dad. He was her sounding board.

Another speaker at the Love Without Life Conference, Sherokee Isle, who lost a baby of her own, wrote a book called *Empty Arms*. She described how her arms ached. Hearing that, Lisa wanted to shout, "Yes!"

"My arms ached. You mean I am not crazy? That was incredibly important for me to hear; I wasn't the only one whose arms physically hurt because there was no child in them."

Another mother said she still had milk.

"Well, I had milk for a long, long time after Betsie died, and that was heartbreaking. It was a reminder every day. But on the other hand, I didn't want it to dry up because then it meant it was really over."

GRANDMA'S DEATH LEADS TO THE SONG

It was ten years later that Lisa wrote her ballad. The song came about when "Ma" died. Lisa was close to her grandmother, and her death brought up a lot of feelings.

"Dad's parents were always 'Ma 'n' Pa.' We were a Kentucky family. Ma was so good to me after Betsie died. She listened to me, and she treated me like a normal person when I wasn't feeling normal at all. I appreciated that. Ma was the best human being I have ever known."

Lisa's grandma had had her own share of pain. She had lost a child, too—her four-year-old son. She buried her parents, her grandparents, her in-laws, two husbands, and all of her brothers and sisters. She was the last of nine brothers and sisters to die.

"And yet she walked through life with so much grace and so much joy. I wanted to be like her when I grew up."

Lisa has fond memories of making "thimble biscuits" with her grandmother when she was small. While they were baking, her grandmother sang to her, talked to her, and listened to her. Ma helped Lisa write her name on a grocery bag.

The night Ma died, the whole family was at her bedside, serenading her as she slipped away. Lisa looked down and saw her grandmother trying to move her lips, and she knew that she could hear them.

It was because of that moment that Lisa was able to write her special song.

"I felt incredibly sad when Ma died, but I kept thinking of how we sang around her hospital bed. Everybody sings in our house, whether we sing well or not does not matter."

Lisa sat down with her guitar and started picking out chords, humming along.

"This tune came into my head, then the words, 'There's a tiny babe in a tiny grave . . . ' appeared. I started scribbling as fast as I could. Somehow it went from being Betsie's song to being Ma's song, too. In the last verse, I say, 'the mother slipped away . . . 'and recite in verse how her children mourned 'with voices joined.'

"That was my tribute to Ma. Getting to sing for her and knowing that she tried to sing back was precious to me. I was able to take that memory and put it in, to honor her for who she was. I was able to tuck my sorrow in a safe place."

> *If you listen near you can almost hear*
> *What the grieving mother cried.*
>
> *Sleep, baby, sleep.*
> *Won't you rest your tired head?*
> *Arms are wrapped around you.*
> *You will soon be fed.*
> *You are wrapped within the Father's love.*

He will hold you now instead.
So, sleep, baby, sleep
Tucked away in God's own bed.

WHY WRITE?

Lisa knows that writing helped her heal, although it did not look that way at first. Even writing letters to acknowledge people's kindness was excruciating.

"Writing thank-you notes afterward was gruesome. I didn't want to see the awful truth in writing. 'Thank you for the lovely gift of flowers on the death'—I couldn't write it—'the death of our daughter.'"

Lisa groans, remembering.

"No, I can't put that in writing, because then I would have to *see* it, and it would be real. It wouldn't be maybe a bad dream, something I was going to wake up from. When you see it in writing, that makes it factual."

And yet, facing reality, as painful as it is, is also healing. Tracy didn't go to the hospital, never saw the baby, and it made it worse for her.

In the beginning, Lisa wrapped herself in make-believe: Perhaps tomorrow, she would wake up and the baby would be fine. She realized that healing would not begin until she got through those days.

"Until you can come out of the desperate fantasy that pretends that this didn't happen, and face the reality that it did, you are stuck. You are stuck in grief, stuck in a place that you can't get past. It's like any other issue where denial comes into play. You can stay in denial and become mentally unstable or you can find your faith and move forward."

Even though she didn't think she could possibly live, wanted to die herself, Lisa had two other children she had to live for.

"In my mind, I didn't have a choice to die. And so I had to find ways of expressing myself that were appropriate, and one of those ways for me was by writing."

Lisa is convinced that grief piles up if you don't handle it head-on.

"What you don't deal with in your twenties, you deal with in your thirties, and what you don't deal with in your thirties, you deal with in your forties, and so on. You just keep on, keep on, keep on until you deal with it."

And writing was a way to deal with the guilt feelings and the "what-ifs" that can tear you apart.

"After Betsie died, I told somebody, The wouldacould-ashoulda's will eat you alive."

She thinks about that and then repeats it for emphasis.

"'The wouldacouldashoulda's will eat you alive,' and that's the truth. If you allow those three to start in your little brain, they are like piranhas; they take *chunks* out of your soul, chunks. Chunks and chunks and chunks until you barely have a soul left.

"That's why I write. I rewrite my chunks and put them back, put the pieces back together."

PLACE OF PEACE

Talking about Betsie's death, even now, all these years later, brings pain, frustration, and hurt.

"And joy, because there was also joy, so much joy."

A friend told Lisa, "It would have been so much easier if you miscarried her."

Lisa's response to that remark was instantaneous and heart-felt.

"Oh no. No, no, no. I had seven days to hold her and touch her and talk to her and get to know her and cherish her; I wouldn't trade those seven days for anything."

She starts to choke up a little, and then laughs nervously.

"It's true, the pain is always there. It hovers. It colors every aspect of my life a little darker shade than it might have been otherwise. But it also makes the color richer, because I have survived. And because she was amazing and she was mine."

Lisa is enjoying most of her 44 years, she says, even if it doesn't sound like it when we talk about the grief aspect.

"I have had such joy in my life. I never dreamed I could have this much happiness, back in the early years when I was still struggling with the Betsie issue. I don't struggle with it anymore.

"I am so blessed. I wake up every day knowing that."

"Sleep Baby Sleep" was published and recorded, and the River Rock Revival Band, Lisa's blue grass and Southern gospel group, sings it regularly in performance.

"We never sing it one time, not once, that somebody doesn't come to us afterward to say, Thank you so much. My grandson died, or, My daughter died, and I have never been able to find any peace in that situation. Your song made me feel better. It does help to put it into words."

APPLY THIS

The Celtic Book of the Dead tells of the Druid midwives: They were not only labor coaches but death coaches. In an ancient ballad, a 12th-century midwife tells how she performed both roles in one day when the baby she delivered died right after birth. She immortalized him in song.

If you have someone dear to you who has passed away, consider writing a song to commemorate that person's life. In the Celtic tradition, these songs could go on for several verses, or be as simple as a haiku, just a few lines.

Considering that this midwife's ballad is still being sung 900 years after that little one's death, the title takes on a deep poignancy: The name of the song is "Please Remember Me."

❧ CHAPTER 4 ❧

Loss of a Job

Exploring the Cave of Her Mind

We met at a booksigning for SARK, the vivacious, outrageous author of *Eat Mangoes Naked* and other similarly titled books. SARK has a way of spreading pixie dust in the air, so that those there catch the festival atmosphere and don't mind standing in long lines to get her autograph.

Jenna waited her turn sitting on the carpeted floor between the bookstore stacks; I sat on the rug beside her, drawn to her happy energy. We started to talk, and before long, she was telling me her story—SARK lines are like that—what happened when she gave up a high-pressured job and was unemployed for half a year. Turns out this lively young woman was a lawyer who worked for the Bill and Melinda Gates Foundation. Turns out her law degree is from Harvard. Pretty high credentials; yet, Jenna told me that, out of work, she went into a pit of depression for six months.

"After I left my job at the Gates Foundation, I had a long dry spell. I felt like a pariah, an absolute loser. I couldn't do the simplest tasks, like make a phone call. I felt this horrible, heavy feeling as though I were moving underwater."

To counteract that mood, Jenna wrote in a journal.

Now this is something I know about losing your job—it can create a sense of loss and self-deprecation. And here is something else I know: writing helps. James Pennebaker of the University of Texas conducted landmark experiments with unemployed people. He was not surprised to find that people who stop working feel both angry and ashamed. What was surprising, though, was that, according to Pennebaker's studies, those who write during this time heal faster and get new jobs more quickly.

But Jenna told me something that made my eyes open wide: During these six dark and fearsome months, she wrote every day in her journal—with *her alternate hand.*

Lucia Capacchione wrote a whole book, *The Power of Your Other Hand,* about what happens when we write with the non-dominant hand, how it releases a part of us that is deep and hidden. Jenna knew nothing of Capacchione, or of Pennebaker. Jenna did instinctively what her heart told her to do—she wrote, and she wrote with her left hand. When pressed for a description, Jenna said that it was a time of such deep introspection and exploration of her soul, it was like "psyche spelunking." She was exploring the cave of her mind.

Jenna and I arranged for a meeting the following week in a neighborhood café. There, Jenna told me the details of her story, and generously shared her unusual journal with me.

"At first, I used my left hand only once in a while, then I did it completely with my left hand. The left hand made it more possible to get in touch with feelings."

Surprisingly, her left-hand script is neater and more legible than her regular, right-hand writing. Jenna has an explanation for this anomaly.

"That's because it is more deliberate—and that's why I was doing it."

RAW EMOTIONS
COMING TO THE SURFACE

Leaving the Gates Foundation, Jenna felt a sense of bereavement. This wasn't what she had expected. She felt adrift.

> It was a beautifully clear and cold day today. Walking over here in the dark and cold and wind it felt like Boston. . . . So much changing, shifting. I am going through another round of what I went through at the end of law school. Another round of surrender, of releasing my little plans and images for how things will be. Grief about the death of those images.

When you lose your job, whether you are fired or you quit, your emotions can run away with you. Jenna found it helped when she acknowledged her feelings rather than fighting them or condemning them.

What does it feel like to be me? Impatient. At people who have let me down. At myself for not working.

Sometimes I feel I could fly to the moon, and other times I feel totally deflated. Barely able to keep on living. . . . if they didn't stink, I'd have a cigarette. Whatever.

I somehow managed to get hugely depressed in the last several hours. Is there a plan to all this time off or is it laziness?

Instead of letting her fears gnaw, in the safety of the page, she comes face to face with them.

I am hard hit by this mood. My frustration is at a high level. I'm sick of myself and my stupid studio. I'd rather be in an office downtown.

I'm not getting anything done, just creating deeper messes and not following through on things I say I'll do, not calling people back, not paying bills, . . . It seems obvious I need to fast or eat better and I tried today but then I ate a vanilla croissant with about 2 lbs of butter in it and now a peanut butter cookie. Good grief, how fast can one girl inhale a cookie?

This whole Seattle world is STUPID and uninteresting.

According to Capacchione, the power of the other hand is that it often lets us express "the disowned and oppressed parts of the self . . . primitive and raw emotions come to the surface."

> Freaking out. On the verge of panicking about how much time off I've had.
>
> I am so worried that I am not going to find work I love. I feel like a planet that broke out of its orbit and now I'm just floating in outer space.
>
> God, I am asking for help here. HELP. I know you are helping. I just can't see it, so show me, let me see.
>
> IS THERE SOMETHING WRONG WITH ME?
>
> God, am I being tested? If this is a test, HELP ME pass it.

As she writes, her words touch a deep part of her, and loosen tears she had been holding back.

> It is raining incredibly hard. I am parked outside the Madison Market. The windows are steamed over from my crying. Listening over and over to Aimee Mann's "It's not going to stop until you wise up." I'm in so much pain. No idea what is next. I've tried so hard to come up with a new career and I still feel stuck.

MINDFULNESS AS
AN ANTIDOTE

When you are depressed, you need an anchor. Alternate-hand writing, because it is deliberate and slow, forces Jenna to be in the present, aware of the now.

"In addition, I always write the date, what time it is, where I am, and what I'm eating."

All of this is important, her way to get her bearings; to say, "Okay, here I am."

peanut butter cookie and coffee for dinner

7:45 pm Bauhaus Café. Chai tea, too peppery and a biscotti. the music is too loud but I'm surrendering.

Here. Now. Anything to establish stability when the world seems in a spin.

now now now listening to an airplane fly overhead. Now feeling my glasses slip down my nose, seeing the fog of their brown plastic frame. Now listening to this silence, full of vibrations, never completely still. Now needing to take a shower. And head downtown.

. . . sitting on the couch, drinking green tea and eating left-over biscuits at 8am on a Saturday morning, listening to Pearl Jam's new CD.

7:50 am North Hill Bakery. Just ate a cinnamon roll, 2 cups of coffee, read the paper, got inspired, now something country/folksy is playing on the radio and there are clouds above but beautiful sunshine coming down over the Olympics and I am remembering why I live here.

Get attuned, be present.

7:45 am. Sunshine outside. Good earth tea. Yellow duvet. Feels like Spring. The sound of a train. Birds.

The deliberation of left-handed writing contributed to Jenna's mindfulness.

"The best antidote to depression is to stay conscious, to appreciate the *what is*.

"That's what I learned with my left-hand. Awareness in the moment, so I don't look back saying, 'Where was I?'"

And sometimes, her left hand reminded her to take care of herself, to, as Jenna put it, "push the reset button."

Yesterday was so incredibly awful [underlined twice], I had to do something to push the reset button and take away all that negative energy. I've spent all day at a Korean spa in Tacoma. I'm there now. I sat in the Mung Wart sauna, had every inch of me scrubbed down, then had a one hour massage, then sauna'ed some more. Now I am

in the restaurant, where I just ordered vege-
tarian yakisoba.

LISTING MAKES IT
CONCRETE, ATTAINABLE

Jenna's left-handed journal has pages and pages of lists.

When the groaning gets too loud, she carefully, meticu-
lously, catalogues good friends, things that make her happy,
people she would invite to a party if she had a party.

"It's just months and months of 'wa, wa, wa,' and then I
write lists of things I am grateful for."

oh yea. I just remembered what I am supposed to do in times like this. Be thankful.
Thanks for my hair, my laughing eyes
and wide smile. I am grateful for:
my perfect mom
my dad's love
my left-handed writing
the sons and daughters I will have someday
my growing yoga practice
friends from high school
my brain
my freedom
my love of words and music
my mental health, most of the time
my love of dance
my exes, such good men
my neighborhood
Seattle

> sunsets
> the spring coming
> my rollerblades
> camping gear
> levi's and clogs
> the fisherman sweater packed away
> this list, truly, is endless

She stops then, and, remembering her own injunction to appreciate *what is*, adds:

> . . . thank you for the chance to be at the
> Gates Foundation. And thank you for this
> time off . . .

Some of Jenna's lists are like debit and credit columns. She laughs at herself when she points them out to me.

"I gave myself 10 points for running that morning, 10 points for everything I did right that day. It added up to 50. Then I *docked* my account: minus 50 for the state of my bank account, minus 10 for eating a chocolate bar; and then to make them even, I thought of something else to add to the plus side."

PRACTICAL
CONCERNS AND MONEY WORRIES

Listing takes the sting out of her worries about money, helping her to get practical and organized. Page after page of figures are headed by questions such as, "How much left?" "How much do I need to live on?" She does the math, calculates insurance costs, let's see, if I earn . . .

Sometimes she panics,

>   deeeeeep breath
>   583.55 OVERDRAWN
>   I just ate an entire chocolate bar based
> on the above information.

She keeps on writing to calm herself down.

>   I keep expecting that if I continue babbling
>   something brilliant will come out.

Just noting facts as statements stops the commotion.

>   So many things up in the air.
>   I'm not as manic as I was last night
>   Job—no kidding. Bring it on.

EXPLORING OPTIONS

Writing slowly, she toys with ideas: should she stay in Seattle, should she move to Taos? Maybe she should be a waitress, or work in juvenile detention.

Her left hand takes ideas and runs with them for awhile:

>   Do I want to be a family lawyer—a baby
>   broker—or do I want to be a political/
>   policy person?

am I a writer? when will I write something for someone else's eyes?

To be a public defender again. Is that really what I want? How law bores me. Totally. Thinking about the public defender's office and being exhausted and having no energy for anything creative. The only thing that makes sense is writing and leading workshops. But on what?

Maybe I should write a column

She takes the time to make plans, spelling out a possible path:

go to LA, make a bunch of $. Get certified to be a yoga teacher. Start teaching yoga one night a week in juvenile detention facility. It's all fine.

Here's another plan: to go to LA for 2 months, make money, come back and work half-time as a lobbyist for the Washington Association of Churches and waitress half-time.

A SHIFT IN PERCEPTION

"Left-handed writing made me realize that there is always a way out. There is always another way of looking at something."

. . . a miracle is a reasonable thing to ask for.
A miracle is a shift in perspective/perception.

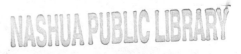

"For me, when I wrote with my opposite hand, it was like a visit with my wise self."

Her wise self told her,

> Keep this space around you. Don't make something happen out of boredom.
>
> what an opportunity you've been given today. A chance to keep the faith when you're not in the mood.

Her wise friend rewrites her horoscope, leading her to clarify her goals.

> My friend's horoscope was great this week. All about daring to ask for what you really want. Mine was about mixing pinstripes and plaids. I think instead I'll ask for what I really want.
>
> I want:
>
> a flexible schedule.
>
> a job I love, where I feel respected and admired and am helping the world.
>
> I want to solve problems on a global scale.
>
> I want to have steady work.
>
> to take care of myself financially
>
> to be loving.
>
> to spread love with everyone that I come in contact with.
>
> to have calm in my eyes and faith in my heart.

so I am done. done with any situation that
asks me to be smaller than I really am.

Something was shifting. Jenna could sense it in the air, and
on the page.

Spring is coming. Time to steam my rug.
Clean and pay bills.
I want to scour my apartment until
there is not one scrap of paper out of place.
Give everything away that I don't need or
love.
Yesterday I put away all my Winter
clothes and got out the Spring/Summer
ones. Had the best night. Folded every pair
of underwear, rearranged furniture. Alpha-
betized my CD's. Heavens.

It is a commonplace of childbirth that the pregnant woman
often gets a neatness urge right before the baby comes. Maybe
some element of that same "nesting instinct" was preparing
Jenna for the new creation in her life. With the flurry of tidiness
came an insight.
"Before, I was so flustered . . . I was in agony. I didn't know
what to do; I thought, 'What is wrong with me?' Then suddenly, it was completely different. I was not agitated anymore."

Yesterday, I heard myself say for probably
the 1200th time, "I'm so confused." But the
thing is, I'm not confused. I know what
kind of connection I'm looking for and

what it feels like. I am not doubtful at all about that.

So I no longer am going to go around saying that I am confused. I am not confused. I am patient and full of faith.

I can't tell you exactly what a new job looks like. I know it feels kind, and I am happy and alive and thankful. And I feel appreciated. And energized.

THE NEW JOB

Action is often an antidote to depression; even a tiny step puts you in forward motion, and may lead to an unpredictable boon.

That is how Jenna finally got her new job.

"I was at an all-time low. Writing in my journal, trying to figure out what to do next. And then I thought, I will do one little thing. I will order this tape from a radio program, of a show that impressed me."

Jenna called California to buy the recording, and wound up talking to the program manager. Several more calls ensued; they shared a common vision. The next thing Jenna knew, they were asking for her resume.

She flew to California for an interview.

It seemed like a fit. The skills she had were what they needed to take the program to the next level.

They invited her to come on board.

She tries on for size what it might sound like, be like to be part of a radio program.

The class I'm taking instead is Radio
Broadcasting. . . .
"You are listening to Jenna B."

WHY IT WORKED

Left-handed writing slowed Jenna down, let her take stock—
and gave her a chance to reinvent herself.

"It was the winter of my life. I wanted everything to be
quiet, which is what left-hand writing did for me."

Writing in this unaccustomed manner changed the rhythm
for this high-powered young attorney.

"To get anything done as a lawyer, I have to operate in a fast
mode—thump, thump, thump. My left hand created a different
pace."

The conscious consideration of such script mimicked the
life message she was trying to learn: slow down, relax, surren-
der the fight.

"It was a time of process and reflecting, rebuilding."

I am unraveling Jenna. To see what's underneath.

For Jenna, left-handed writing changed her cadence at a
time in her life when she needed to be introspective. Once she
was back in the work world, she could hardly imagine that
painstaking tempo, had no attraction to it. Left-handed writing
now seems foreign to her. Once it was the most natural thing,
the only thing.

"Everything is moving so fast now that I have no time to explore the inner landscape. When I was doing it, I became quite good at using the left hand to write; now I am impatient with it and have gone back to right-hand writing."

Through her alternate-hand writing, though, Jenna discovered values that she plans to incorporate into her life.

> Remember how I used to feel? Just craving time off . . . I have had so much time off. And I wonder if it will all melt away now that I am working again, or if I can hold on to this. What is this? a yoga practice, a deep faith, a clean house. Time with friends, journal writing. These are meaningful and enriching.

Left-handed writing did for Jenna exactly what she first asked from it—to shift her perspective, to see the possibilities, to recognize the potential, the miracles all around—the open doors where the shut one was.

> I feel STRONG when I think about doing this broadcasting job in California. Life is long—God willing—and there is time to do many jobs.

APPLY THIS

I met a young man named Montana who is head mechanic at a bike shop. He uses a typewriter instead of a computer. He likes the fact that his antiquated Smith-Corona creates a deliberate handicap to make him more thoughtful. Montana told me how Samuel Beckett, the Nobel Prize–winning Irish dramatist, wrote *Waiting for Godot* in French, and then translated it back into English. Working first in a second language forced the playwright to choose words carefully.

Likewise, the disconcerting awkwardness of writing with the unschooled hand changes the rules, thwarts the expected response, the supposed correct way.

Try it, even if it seems odd at first and off-putting. It may help you be more centered, and teach you to look at the world with new eyes.

❧ CHAPTER 5 ❧

Discernment

Holding Your Sorrow
and Your Joy Together

I called Jack Kennedy, a former priest living in Portland, Oregon, when I heard that he leads groups through Discernment, a decision-making process based on *The Spiritual Exercises* of Ignatius of Loyola, the founder of the Jesuit Order. Jack could hardly contain his enthusiasm for this simple yet stunning formula that even now, 550 years after the death of Ignatius, continues to enrich people's lives.

I have studied Discernment, and lived by its principles for many years, but I had yet to find anyone who could articulate it as brilliantly and succinctly as Jack Kennedy. He has distilled centuries of application and scholarship into accessible language and format.

The *Exercises* of Ignatius are a great boon to people in pain, because Ignatius teaches how to hold your sorrow and joy together, and to learn from strong feelings. When you combine this practice with writing, an amazing transformation takes place. You will find the path that is best for you, and end up following your heart. You will move, in Ignatian terms, from desolation to consolation, from a place of agony to a place of peace.

Jack fell in love with Ignatius, and with the exercises and rules or guidelines of Discernment.

"They were my passion, who knows why? I believe for our country today if people lived out Discernment, it would invite us back to being who we were called to be."

Ignatius bids you reflect on your own experience, and to ask yourself tenderly, What is this experience doing to me? Discernment is a tool that gives you clarity in the midst of chaos.

The norms of Discernment are universal, but their application is unique. Two people with exactly the same data can arrive at different decisions. And each of them have uncovered what is best for him or her.

"Ignatian Discernment," says Jack, "has been part of my life. Probably the most Jesuit thing I ever did, the most Ignatian thing, was to leave the Jesuits. I had been helping people to discern for years and I never owned up to trusting for myself. When I did, I knew in faith that God was inviting me to go."

"SPIRIT": A STIRRING INSIDE

The Exercises are based on what is going on inside you. In the most basic language, Ignatius says, "Ask for what you desire."

How do you know what you desire in life? Well, the first step is to pay attention to what attracts you and what repulses you.

Jack looks for what ignites people.

"When I see that spark, they are in touch with an inner passion. I tell them, Sit in that space where you live. When you watch a show on Bosnia, where do you experience your response to that? That's where you live. Can you be aware of it, without judging it? Or if you're watching Michelle Kwan skate, what goes on in you?"

If something makes you cry, "Track back your tears to find out where they are welling up from."

Notice your interior movements: "That's not necessarily getting from a to b, but a stirring inside."

One way to focus your awareness on what is moving inside of you is to draw a picture of your heart, and pencil inside of it whatever you are feeling at this precise moment.

Go ahead and do this for yourself right now.

List everything you are holding in your heart today without condemning or hiding any of it. Include everything. It is all part of who you are at this moment. Your heart might look something like this.

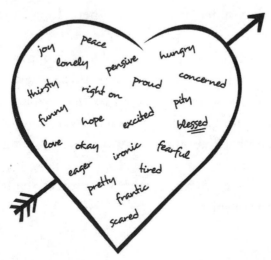

Jack says that when he does this exercise with a group, they are initially surprised at what comes out of the tip of their pen. They didn't know how much was in their heart.

Pick one or two of the strongest feelings, and explore them further in writing. Keep in mind that there are no "bad" feelings or "good" feelings; everything in your heart is part of who you are. When you respect all aspects of your own humanity, then your choices will be shaped by what you are about, rather than dictated by the "shoulds" that get imposed on you from the outside.

Movement of spirit is not an esoteric concept; Jack brings it down to earth.

"We say, 'My spirits are down' or 'I am in high spirits today,' or we might use the phrase in describing someone else, 'She is a spirited woman.'"

Stop and think about what is behind those expressions.

"Whatever causes your spirit to be happy and dancing, and whatever leads your spirits to droop—that is the affective life."

Write down what you desire, and then go beyond what you want to have happen and identify underneath the feelings driving that goal.

"Where do you feel frustration, where do you feel hope? In what part of your body, where within you, do you experience that desire? What is going on there? How strong is it?"

Writing it out helps you reply to these questions, even if you do not know when you begin to write what you want to say. Keep on writing, and let the pen answer for you.

Jack is emphatic about the importance of being connected to your feelings.

"You need to be in touch with your affective life to discern the movement of spirit."

CONSOLATION AND DESOLATION

Feelings are not right or wrong, but they can provide a clue to what makes you tick. Ignatius uses the terms "consolation" and "desolation" to describe the indicators that let you know whether or not you are on the path that is meant for you.

In the book *Freedom*, part of the *Take and Receive* series, Jacqueline Syrup Bergan and S. Marie Schwan list typical telltale signs of consolation: "feelings of harmony, peace and contentment." Conversely, in desolation, be on the lookout for "feelings of fear, anxiety, heaviness, restlessness" as well as "discouragement, alienation, dryness, and lack of fervor."

The central consideration in Discernment, however, is not just what are you feeling, but where is that feeling coming from, and what is it moving you toward? It is not as simple as saying, Go with what makes you happy, avoid what depresses you. Sometimes what makes you sad has a message for you, if you will be patient enough to listen for it.

You can be sad, and still be in consolation.

Jack explains, "Desolation is anything that leads to lack of faith, hope, or love; anything that causes turmoil of spirit, or is de-energizing. Consolation can be found in something painful, if it is life-giving and meaningful.

"The question I always ask is, Is this feeling opening me up to being more fully human in some way?"

A drug addict going through withdrawal in a treatment program, for example, is in great pain.

"He knows that if he embraces his sadness and loss instead of burying it, or numbing himself, he has a better chance staying off drugs."

When Jan's baby died, the sight of small salt-water sandals made her cry.

"Moments like that are part of consolation. She is grieving the loss of her daughter, honoring how sensitive and deep a woman she is. That is rich. That is the spirit groaning in her.

"It is humanizing to feel your sadness. It opens you up to your own compassion and love and sense of loss."

Even anger can be consolation.

"Anger is an honest emotion. It says there's something wrong with this picture. It moves us to justice."

Stay with a feeling when you don't immediately know the source of it.

Jack tells of a time he broke down crying in front of his director because he was so sad. He did not know where the tears were coming from.

"The guy was smart enough to direct me to go and be with my sadness for the day."

Being with it opened Jack up to what his sadness was about.

"I missed having a family, and I was grieving. I was acting out of that. I was able to mourn it, and then feel my joy also."

That was consolation.

THE EXAMEN: THE END OF THE DAY

Dennis, Sheila, and Matthew Linn, in their lovely book *Sleeping with Bread,* suggest a simplified version of what Ignatius called the Examen. The Examen is a daily exercise taking stock of your spirit. Because it heightens your awareness of who you are (it is sometimes called the Awareness Examen) and what you are drawn to, the Examen is the underpinning of Ignatian Discernment. It is a reckoning, at the end of the day, of the darkness and light in your life, and the times when you most felt energy and excitement, or conversely, deflation and inertia.

The Linns encourage you to reflect on the moments throughout your day for which, looking back, you were the most, and the least, grateful. What part of your day would you relive if you could, and which rather not? They invite you to relish the periods when you felt the most alive, and consider what about the other moments might have made them difficult. Don't try to change or fix those experiences, they advise, just hold them gently.

The Examen works best when you do it in writing. It could be as simple as jotting down your feelings in a little memo book, or exploring your feelings at greater length in a journal.

If you did nothing more than this, to spend some time in the evening reflecting in writing on the high and the low points of your day, it would contribute immeasurably to the richness of your existence, your awareness of who you are. This one little exercise could revolutionize your life.

Jack suggests you do the Examen for a month, say, around a particular issue.

"Then go back and look for the patterns of freedom, the patterns of hope, patterns of depression, until you get a sense of what you might choose to do—which one seems more life-giving than the other."

Writing the examen gives you a record. When you read it over, you will see some feelings coming up again and again. You might be surprised to see that every time you considered a certain course of action, you got optimistic, or maybe you were scared, but did not realize it came up so often.

Pay attention. These repetitions are telling you something about your life. The Awareness Examen moves you toward those moments that set you on fire and tracks what happens when you ignore or disregard them.

"All a sudden, a door is open. You are being invited, or called."

Ignatius himself carried a little notebook in his pocket and noted the direction of his life. A soldier in the Spanish Army, he was living a dissolute existence, and trying to sort it out.

"He set up the Discernment process because of his own worldliness, womanizing, and drinking. He had to reflect on his own experience."

THE LISTENING PART

Jack outlines the three prerequisites for Discernment:

"First, you are in touch with your interior life. Second, you can articulate that, express what is going on inside. Third, and perhaps the toughest, is an attitude of indifference."

Indifference is not passive; it does not mean that you do not care; it means you care deeply, but you are willing to let go of being right. It means you are willing to trust your story to another individual and allow him or her to feed back to you what they hear.

"Ignatius said if it's in the dark, an important part of Discernment is to bring it into the light to somebody with whom you feel safe."

Invite that person to hold your experience with you, out in the light together, tenderly; not to solve it, but to play it back and explore with you what shuts you down, what moves you to a fuller life, even if it frightens you. Ask them to listen without giving advice, without judging, without trying to fix it.

"When I listen in this way, I listen for the longing, the passion. I reflect it back. I ask, If you held that energy, would it lead you to choose to do this, rather than that? And then I look at their historical context. If the spirit is working in them, the spirit will already show up in the ways they have committed themselves in the past."

When someone listens to you in this total way, you can sense the compassion and the love coming back to you.

"That is an incredible feeling, both freeing and healing."

FIVE STEPS TO PROBLEM SOLVING

There are many models based on Ignatius's approach. The chief components common to all of them include:

1. gathering external evidence
2. examining internal feelings
3. looking at blocks or attachments
4. making a provisional decision
5. confirming the final choice

As an example of Discernment in action, Jack graciously shared with me his own process in the radically life-changing decision he made to leave the Jesuit Order after 32 years as a priest.

"This is my story. Choosing to leave the priesthood was a huge decision for me. It took me four years to resolve, because it was not clear. I came up with all the reasons to stay and all the reasons to go, and they were so good on both sides. I was caught; I felt trapped.

"I finally had to trust."

(1) Gathering External Evidence

Bergan and Schwan present several lines of inquiry to consider at this preparatory stage. You might question how the idea originated, what costs are involved, what sacrifices you and the people affected by this decision might have to make. You need to be honest about the risks involved.

Bring together as much information as possible, collect documents, research the topic on both sides thoroughly, talk with experts, read whatever you can get your hands on.

Jack did this, and then he put his vocation in the context of his life.

It is a fact that Jack entered the Jesuits right out of high school. He says that it was like going directly from home to another form of home.

"In a way, I never got out on my own."

Jack concedes that for some people, that would not be a problem.

"For me, I had not developed socially or looked at my options in terms of what God might be calling me to. I jumped too fast."

Had he gotten married at 18, he might have faced the same dilemma years later.

"I'm not sure I wouldn't have ended up having to leave the marriage because I would have needed to find me, to do that piece of individuation which I never got to do in my early twenties. Inevitably, I came to the point where I needed to do that in order for me to be healthy in my life. "

Yet he was grappling with another reality, the fact that he had taken a vow. He felt bound by that. Would it be wrong to disregard it?

"I said yes forever; can you say yes forever?"

Answering that question was part of his growing-up process.

After struggling with it for a long time, he realized, "I wasn't saying no to anything. I was saying a bigger yes, and it had to do with my finally owning my own adulthood. I had let myself stay a kid for so long."

Looking candidly at his life, he saw the disproportion. He was hiding behind his service to others.

He was a good minister, loving and compassionate, but he never slowed down enough to think.

"I was a workaholic. When I tried to put a balance in my life, there was room to breathe. And that was when I got in touch with my desolation. I said yes to everything, because I would not face my own pain."

He came to a stunning conclusion.

"People find coping mechanisms when they live with something for a long time, and if they stay numb enough they can do it."

Doing the daily examen would not allow him to live on that level any longer. He could no longer stay numb. He had to face his feelings and discern what they were telling him.

(2) Examining Interior Feelings

"The examen gives me information about myself. I want to honor that information when I make a choice."

Jack started charting his interior feelings around the priesthood.

"I needed to jot down affectively where my darkness and discouragement was, and where I felt alive and hopeful. Part of Discernment is recognizing where I experience life. Not where

I *wish* I experienced it, or *should* experience it, but where I *do*. And if I own that, I step out of my denial, there is another chance for life in that."

Jack felt most fully alive and human when he was with the people in his congregation.

"When I trusted those aspects and put them down on paper, when I shared them with my therapist and my spiritual director, it was freeing."

In the rectory, he felt a sense of isolation.

"Living in an all-male structure wound up feeling very desolate to me. I felt de-energized. That is not a judgment on the lifestyle; it was just what went on inside of me when I tried to live that lifestyle. I loved my brothers, the individuals I lived with, very much, but I am emotionally dead when I continue to live with a whole group of men. I was shut down and taking it out on people."

When a man leaves the priesthood, people assume it is because of celibacy. What was driving Jack was not sexuality in that narrow sense.

"It was more that there was not even the possibility of a long-term committed relationship with a woman that was deadening to me. It did not have to happen to me, I just needed to live in that possibility and freedom."

(3) Looking at Blocks or Attachments

As you move forward in your decision-making, consider the blocks that stand in your way, and what they tell you about your way of thinking. Bergan and Schwan, for example, suggest that you reflect on the part that prestige plays in your indecisiveness, or perhaps you are driven by an "overconcern for success or achievement" or locked into staying in a certain geographic location. Such considerations can impede your freedom to make a clear choice.

When you are invited to do something, and your first response is "No way," challenge yourself to ask, Where did that "No" come from? Maybe it came from fear or your own self-talk rather than a legitimate refusal. Explore that a little bit, learn more of what caused that knee-jerk reaction. Sit with it, write about it, and it will tell you something about the blocks that are holding you back, perhaps in other areas of your life as well.

For Jack the first block was economic.

"That was a biggie I came right up against."

As a priest, he was living a life where all his needs were taken care of by his community.

"I did not own one thing, and all of a sudden, I am wondering how am I going to make money? I am 50 years old; I never tried to look for work; I didn't have any marketable skills. Can I provide for myself? Where am I going to live? How am I going to pay my rent? That was huge for me."

Tied in with that was the darkness that rose up around security.

"If I stayed a priest, I had a cemetery plot all picked out for me; I had an infirmary to go to when I was sick; there was no limit to my health care."

Out in the world by himself, he would have to figure out medical benefits and worry about retirement.

Then there was the matter of respect. People looked up to him; even his own mom and dad were proud of him for being a priest.

He feared that leaving the priesthood would let others down.

"It would be discouraging to my friends who are other Jesuits, and to all the lay people I had worked with for so many years. I felt guilty."

But Jack knew from years of teaching others that he could not allow this to be a factor. How many times he had said to them what he now told himself:

"Do not let guilt decide for you. Being guilty and feeling guilty are two different things."

Finally, he followed his own advice.

"I let go of all the reasons, and just paid attention to what was life-giving, what enlivened my spirit, and then what deadened me inside, made me irritable and cranky, and shut me off from people."

Then it became crystal clear to him what he needed to say yes to.

"And it was scaring the hell out of me: I needed to leave the Order."

Or at least, try leaving it on for size and see if that was what was right.

(4) Provisional Decision

My cousin Mary Edna had a game she played with me growing up, whenever I was torn making up my mind between two attractive options. She would challenge me to pick either one, and then, fast, test my response in my stomach to that choice. Little did we know, at an early age, we were working in the Ignatian tradition. One of the more revealing aspects of Ignatian Discernment is the use of the provisional decision and what it tells you about yourself.

Pick one: Stay where you are, and live with the present circumstances, or make the leap and do something different.

"Lean in to each decision: Which one seems to have a better chance of something life-giving or something hopeful, even if you are fearful; and which one sounds like it will continue to reinforce discouragement? Look for darkness and light, and the spirit in that. Where does the spirit have the chance of coming to live and where does it not?"

Ignatius suggests here that you write out both the advantages and the disadvantages of each side, letting your reason help you determine which way you are leaning.

In place of Ignatius's chart, I prefer at this point in the process to substitute Edward de Bono's eye-opening "PMI." In his book, *de Bono's Thinking Course* he explains this quick and clever device.

Write the letters, P, M, I down the side of the page.

The P stands for Plus, the M is Minus, and the I is Interesting.

Now make up your mind, one way or the other, and then write out, fast and furiously, the thoughts around that decision in the three categories, as though it were a done deal. Do it rapidly, without stopping to consider. The plus, the minus, the interesting. Write down whatever comes to mind, even if it seems absurd or irrelevant. Three minutes.

And then switch sides. And do another PMI.

I will / I won't. Three minutes for each.

According to de Bono, the PMI is much more than a pro/con chart, which is useful for weighing different sides in a judgement evaluation. The PMI, on the other hand, can shift your perception of a problem. When you, in his phrase, "do a PMI," it is not a matter of numerical density but rather resonance. One Minus item could negate ten Pluses if that one Minus spoke strongly to you. Or one Plus can jump off the page: it speaks to your spirit—and you know, that's it, That's the choice.

De Bono has shown time and again, whether working with third graders or Olympic planning committees, that the PMI can change minds in three minutes, especially when people go into the exercise already convinced of the answer, already decided on a situation, absolutely dead-sure that they are right. The PMI forces you to think of other options when you might have closed the door to them.

I use the PMI regularly, for everything from deciding whether or not to attend an all-day opera seminar to exploring the possibilities of applying for a community college position teaching medieval literature. De Bono's method is one of my favorite writing tools. It helps break the tie in provisional decision making. (For examples, see the Appendix.)

For Jack, the provisional decision-making step spanned four years. He was given a leave of absence for three years, then he went back in for one year. During both periods, he carefully monitored his feelings of desolation and consolation until his answer was absolute. At the end of the fourth year, he left the priesthood for good.

(5) Confirming the Final Choice

After you make a final decision, look for external and internal signs of validation.

Bergan and Schwan tell us some validating internal signs might be peace and harmony; external signs are circumstances supporting your choice, doors opening, help available.

For Jack the latter came from former parishioners.

"When I left, people in that parish called up and offered me a place to live. I have been totally embraced by this group of people I used to say Mass for."

He counts on their support today.

"I have such a safety net in friends. I couldn't end up on the street if I wanted to, they would come down there and collect me."

As for internal confirmation, Jack had a tremendous sense of peace. He differentiates between peace and relief.

"You can think you are peaceful because you are so relieved to have made a decision. I felt more than that. It was a quiet sense of peace, like drop of water on a sponge. It fit; it was right, and it did not matter if I had a stroke the next day or if I didn't find work."

But he admits trying to find a job was tough. He applied to drive a pizza truck, but at first it seemed nobody would hire him.

"There is no harder work than looking for work. I spent three days in the fetal position in my bed because I was so scared to even look for work. God, that is hard on the self-esteem."

Even though he was petrified, that fear was consolation, because he knew that going through it was life-giving.

Today he has a job he enjoys, working as a paid administrator for a volunteer organization, but in the beginning, he painted houses, he cleaned motel rooms—and he had an epiphany. There was consolation in menial labor.

"I thought to myself, You know, I may never earn a huge salary, but I can earn enough to get through the day. I can earn $6 or $7 an hour, and I will always be able to do that if I have my health. And I'm okay.

"So I was getting confirmed in just doing the basic 'chop wood, carry water' and I was finding out I liked it."

And he was fine. For the first time in a long time, he felt at home with himself.

"And I was at peace with God; I was at peace with the Jesuits; I was at peace with the world."

Leaving the priesthood was a leap of faith.

"Pretty hard to do, actually. But I never looked back. I am so damn happy. I really am."

WHY WRITE?

Writing is a perfect way of getting both your thoughts and your feelings into the light.

Jack says he tells people, "'Let your pen go, don't pay attention or try to control it, just let it rip.' It is amazing what comes out. Then when they read back what they wrote, they say, 'God, I didn't know I felt that deeply.' It starts to give them a sense of hope: Maybe they have the energy to deal with whatever the problem is."

When you write your thoughts and feelings, there is something deep and primal happening. Jack uses a biblical image to articulate the profundity and sacredness of it.

"The Hebrew word *dabar* is an infinitive action word. When God created the world, he spoke into the void: *dabar*. How do I put this? If I keep it inside of me, it never becomes reality—but if I speak it out, if I proclaim it, if I yell into the void, or if I write it onto the paper, it takes on life. If I don't get it out on the page, it's not born. If I can put it down, I can feel it. I can let it flow out of me into the world. I'm talking about discovering what's going on inside me. I let it go out of me so that it can be reflected."

Writing brings a fullness to ideas which holding them in your mind alone will never accomplish. Because when you write something down, it speaks back to you.

"You go back and read what you wrote, and sometimes things hit you that you never got out of it before, that you never knew you knew."

Psychologists call this "knowing without knowing," when you know, but do not know you know.

"You see it on the page and say, 'My God, did I write that? Look at that. I wrote that down ten times, and I did not realize what was going on in me.'"

Sometimes in your writing, you come to an insight you think you just arrived at. You forget what you wrote months earlier. You finally realize a key connection in your life, a stunning perception that feels brand new and brilliant; light bulbs are popping. And then, looking back in an old journal, you are startled to find that you actually came to the *very same* conclusion, say, a year ago.

Jack has an explanation for this phenomenon.

"Figuring it out is not living it out. When you live into it, then it takes on a reality you don't forget."

It is tempting to look for solutions when you write. Jack suggests a different mentality.

"I tell people, instead of looking for an answer, just jot down your experience, capture your experience in writing."

Then you can flip back through it like a photo album, and recall and relive things.

"Writing is not just a record of the past. Let your writing be a way of supporting you in living out something."

That is exactly what Jan learned. Rereading the journals of Justine's death gave her the courage to live her life today. Later you will meet Debra, and Mike. Writing kept Debra from going back to an abusive husband. And, after living through Vietnam, writing helped Mike, and now his friends and family understand who he is today, and why he loves to draw. Their writing was not just a record of the past, but it supports them in living out the present.

When you read a letter from a friend, it is not like reading a history text, it is like reading one person's heart. Writing in a journal or a notebook or even on a pad of paper is like a letter to yourself.

"You get to read what is going on in your own heart; and it speaks back to you," says Jack.

"It is almost as though you get a language for how you have lived, to put a language on what you already know. That is how it speaks back to you."

APPLY THIS

Track, at the end of the day, what brought you light, and what made you sad or put you down. It can be as quick as marking little up ⇑ or down ⇓ arrows next to a list of the day's activities.

When you are making an important decision, follow the five steps outlined above, then make a "provisional decision." Use de Bono's PMI to test its rightness for you. Pay attention to feelings of "desolation" and "consolation."

Let your writing speak back to you.

CHAPTER 6

September 11, 2001

Finding Comfort in the Familiar

Though he now lives in Seattle, Tim has a special connection to lower Manhattan. He grew up in New Jersey, and lived and worked in New York City.

The journal he shared with me begins in April of 2001. He is sitting on the grass in Central Park—frisbee players, cyclists, runners all around him—trying to come to grips with his disappointment because he didn't get the position he had just applied for, with Prudential Securities. He was interviewed for four hours. The job was in the World Trade Center.

There was the possibility of employment on the West Coast.

"My cousin John told me, 'Dude, you don't have to live in New York to make money. You can live anywhere and make money.' That's all I needed to hear. 'Why don't you go work on one of Paul Allen's yachts?'"

> Sheep Meadow, Central Park. I am confused these days about everything. I try to keep in mind what Ed Powers, my junior year in high school civics teacher said: "Confusion is a wonderful thing. Don't be afraid of it." That man has lived some life to come up with that simple, yet profound statement.
>
> I'm so tired and so much is going on; four hour interviews at Prudential, talking with people at Microsoft. My living situation is not definite. It's as if I am trying to get settled in my own skin. New York? Seattle?

He had some huge choices to make.

> I am in limbo for the moment—decisions about living, working, and relationships. I am at a strange point in my life, in-between jobs, in-between places to live, there is this restless angst in me.

Could Seattle cure his restlessness, or was that feeling just part of being 20something?

> If there wasn't this unsettledness and excitement in the last months of my 26th year, I suppose life would be boring.
> The 20's sure are an up and down trip. The peaks and valleys begin to level out, or so I've been told. I'm hoping. I can only live

through my 20's once. If I had to do it twice
it would kill me.

Over the next few months, Tim constantly returns to his
journal and to New York's 840-acre urban sanctuary to sort
through his discouragement and disorder. His life seems a jumble, his journal the one constant.

> Central Park, Great Lawn, looking at
> people around me and wondering, are all
> these people as lost as I am, or am I a special
> breed? I'm sure they're all equally lost in
> one way, shape, or form. I just happen to be
> lost in several ways, shapes and forms.

Even though the job situation on the West Coast was still
uncertain, Tim decided to move to Seattle.

> Packed up my life yesterday and shipped it
> to the other coast. 22 boxes.
>   I am presently waiting to hear whether I
> got a job from the beast Microsoft. I can remember writing a long time ago in my ideological college days how pretty soon everyone was going to be working for Bill Gates.
> And now here I am, waiting on a job from
> the man.

He was eager for a change, but he was going to miss the
excitement of New York.

> I am in the heart of New York City on a
> beautiful rooftop on the Upper West Side.

All of Manhattan is around me. Last night I
was on Malcolm Forbes's yacht, the *High-
lander,* drinking bourbon.

The beat never stops in NYC. The electric-
ity is always around you, everything inten-
sified. The mind never rests. Constant pul-
sating energy.

Summer nights in New York City rooftops.
As magical as this New York City skyscape
is, I am ready for something else.

It is early July,

Here I am on a rooftop in Manhattan, about
to move cross-country. I am 11 days away
from my 27th birthday, three days away
from making the biggest move of my life.

COMING TO SEATTLE

On the flight to Seattle, he was feeling poetic. Little did he realize the luxury of traveling with so much baggage.

This is not the first time I have wholeheartedly entered the western night, however last
time I was driving into it. Tonight I am
aboard the Jet Blue Flight #83, armed with
five massive bags and one guitar in the
cargo hold, two carry-ons above me, and
one at my feet. How should I feel right

now? I am launching myself headlong into
the unknown carrying only a dream.

For a fellow who frequently found an oasis in Central Park,
it is not surprising that Tim is drawn immediately to the natural
beauty of the Cascade Mountains. For him, the grandeur lifted
his spirits and seemed a metaphor of what the West could be for
him, of limitlessness.

> The Manhattan skyline is impressive, and
> certainly a testament to a man's curiosity and
> aspirations, but it can't compete with Mother
> Nature's structure of the Pacific Northwest.
>
> I am sitting before Mount Rainier near
> Paradise base camp. In the heart of Mt.
> Rainier National Park. It is awe-inspiring.
>
> My vision of heaven is here. Heaven is
> walking through mountain canyons on pine
> needle paths. Every so often there are
> breathtaking vistas and you are filled with
> Divine knowledge.
>
> Sometimes what sounds like voices of
> angels sing your favorite song, echoing
> throughout the canyon.

"In the West, the possibilities seem endless. Life feels good
out here."

GETTING INTO THE SCENE

Soon, Tim assimilates into the Seattle scene, even learns the
proper way to order steamed milk and espresso.

I'm sitting in downtown Seattle and I just
scored some junk—the caffe latte. When the
man behind the counter asked me what size I
wanted, I panicked and ordered a medium. I
should have known: Grande, grande, grande.
I'll learn.

Tim was still checking things out at Microsoft, meeting with
people there, and whenever he could, he got near water.

Discovery Park on Puget Sound, Seattle,
Washington. The water has a way of pacify-
ing me. I've discovered that I like living by
the water and seeing the mountains. It's inspiring and peaceful.
   I'm still holding onto New York ten-
dencies. The main difference is that my
mind is open to potential. I feel hope for the
first time in a long time.

One night, he and his roommates, Ben and Jessica, rented a
video of *Sex in the City*. It made him homesick.

For the first time, seeing that, I really
missed New York. But I think it was just
missing out on being in on all that action. It
really is the heartbeat.

Seattle offered a chance for a fresh start, and a different kind
of adventure.

There is a frontiersman attitude about the
West. You move out here and arrive with

the 49ers spirit. Hope, possibility and the
crazy notion that you could strike it rich.

The action in the Pacific Northwest may not be as large-
scale and fast-paced as the East, but there are still a lot of things
to do with your friends. In early September, Tim goes to a famous festival at the Seattle Center, Seattle's 74-acre version of
Central Park. The festival is named after the umbrella, the symbol of Seattle's fabled rainfall.

> Monday Labor Day was a blast. I went with
> Nancy to Bumbershoot. . . I spent almost
> the entire weekend at Bumbershoot seeing
> countless bands. It made me want to play or
> be part of music.

Less than two weeks later, Tim would be back at Seattle
Center for more somber reasons, and the music would be
solemn Tibetan drumming, not rock bands. And there would
be no smiles. And no dancing. Just as many people, maybe
more, but silence, no sound of conversation or laughter.

SEPTEMBER 11TH

Tim could not write on September 11th. He tried, but nothing
came out. It was the following day, September 12th, that he
wrote a play-by-play of the day before.

"I wanted to lay it out as a record. Some of it is complete
thoughts, other parts just jotting down what was going through
my mind."

It was 6:30 in the morning, Pacific Time. Tim was in bed
when the phone rang.

Who is calling me at 630 in the morning? I
ignored it.

The phone rang again 15 min later and I
thought nobody calls that early in the morning twice.

"Phone calls at that hour are never good news, and I immediately listened to the message, thinking of my family."

. . . expecting bad news about my father, I
checked the answering machine.

It was a friend of my roommate's from
Connecticut. He said, Turn on the TV. An
airplane just crashed into the Twin Towers.

"Same as everyone, I thought it was a biplane flying off the
river, and then I turned the news on . . .

"'What tha?' I was horrified."

Tim immediately woke up his roommates, Ben and Jess.

"They came running in, we stood there like this. . ." his
mouth drops open "and then, all of a sudden, all of a sudden. . ." his voice chokes up ". . . the . . . a plane hits the Pentagon and then another plane hits and then we . . . we . . . I was
afraid. I didn't know what to do."

We all just stood there and stared at the TV
dumbfounded. We were in shock and said
nothing.

Tim was concerned about his family, especially his sister,
who regularly goes into New York and meets with designers.

"I didn't know if she was going in that day or whatnot. Cell phones were down."

He felt frantic. He left messages everywhere.

"'Please. Call me when you get this.'"

Ben's father sometimes conducted business in the World Trade Center. Ben tried to reach him, but to no avail.

Finally after what seemed like an eternity, Ben reached his father, who was in his office in Exchange Place, the tallest office building in New Jersey, directly across from the World Trade Center.

As they spoke to each other, the first building went down.

> Ben's father simply said, "Oh my God, it's going down." Ben's father watched it live and in person and we watched it live on television. There wasn't much to say.
>
> Meanwhile, every few minutes a new report came in, as a plane crashed into the Pentagon, and another in rural Pennsylvania.
>
> We all sat on eggshells.

Ben had an interview that morning, and he didn't know what to do about it. Tim tried to persuade him to stay home.

"I told him, 'Don't go, don't leave the house. Who knows what the hell is going to happen?'"

Not knowing how else to handle it, Ben decided to go.

"He said, 'I gotta go. I gotta get out of here.'"

"His girlfriend offered to go with him and I was hoping she didn't.

"Jess asked, Do you want me to go with you? Silently I was thinking, 'God, please don't go, don't leave me alone.'"

. . . thank God she didn't go. I was afraid to
be alone.

Ben left for the interview. After a while, Jess and Tim
couldn't bear to watch the relentless images anymore. They had
to get out. Tim wanted to be near water.

> We were both disgusted with the images on
> TV, so we went for a walk down to Lake
> Washington and sat more or less in silence.
> On the way there, and on the way home, it
> was all anybody could talk about. Already
> neighbors were out on the porch saying
> what a terrible thing this was.

"All I could think was, I can't believe what is going on in
New York right now."

The picture in Madison Park felt out of kilter.

"Some guy was playing with his kid. The guy had ear-
phones on; we all knew what he was listening to.

"It was the most beautiful surreal scene. Here we were by
the lake and the mountains, and in New York, people were running for their lives and dying . . . "

His voice trails off, and there is a moment of absolute quiet
between us. It is too hard to continue.

> Ben came home awhile later and we all sat
> around the television basically speechless all
> day as images of horror and terror that will
> never escape us came across the screen. It
> was the day when all else changed in the

world. From that day on nothing is or will ever be the same.

That night two friends came over, and Ben's sister.

We had a Greek salad together, drank some beers, and watched the news. Some of us could watch, others were out on the porch.

Ben's sister and I slept in bed together and held each other tight. I, a solitary person, an introvert for the most part, was scared to be alone.

PERSONAL STORIES

Tim got an E-mail from his friend Frost, sent at noon PST.

"He told me the most incredible story. He ran to the bottom of Manhattan, to the lighthouse there, and they wouldn't open the doors because they were afraid that everyone would get crushed to death.

"So he had to rip down a fence. He was there when the clouds came over, the blackest black he has ever seen. 'This is it, I'm going to die.' Then after five minutes, it cleared."

Frost continued running, up the FDR Drive and across the Brooklyn Bridge.

"He was walking fast across the Brooklyn Bridge when a car stopped. Everyone freaked out; they thought someone had a car bomb and was planning to blow up the bridge."

Frost showed up at his friend's apartment in Brooklyn and E-mailed Tim. His mom and dad live near Seattle, and he couldn't reach them.

"'Please contact my parents in Bainbridge Island, tell them I am alive and all right.'

"He told me he was like those people you saw on TV, covered in gray."

Tim stops, considering, trying to take it all in.

"I can't even imagine. I don't know how you can live through that."

There were the incredible stories of friends who worked in the Twin Towers who were spared.

"Two of my friends were late for work; they walked out of the subway, and looked up to see the plane hit.

"Another guy I know went to a Giants game the night before and got blasted. He woke up with a hangover, and he didn't go to work Tuesday morning."

Tim had a close friend, a college classmate, who didn't make it.

Tim found out about Sean watching TV.

"I saw his sister on the news, crying, walking around in shock, holding the sign 'Please, if you see my brother. . . .'

"I thought to myself, 'That looks like Stephanie Lugano,' and just then, her name flashed across the bottom of the screen.

"Oh. My. God."

Later, Tim read an article about Sean in the *Boston Herald*, and he was dead. He worked on the 88th floor of Tower Two. He was 28 years old.

DAY THREE: SLEEP, CLEAN, PONDER

On the third day, Tim slept on and off because he had had so much trouble sleeping the two nights before.

> News, sleep, News, sleep. And then I did
> what I always do to clear my head, I cleaned.

During the cleaning, the gravity of the situation began to hit him.

> While this is day three and I'm still in shock, a bit of the shock wore off, and I have begun to feel grief, fear, and anger. I have not been able to let that grief go.
>
> I've tried not to watch TV today. I called friends, E-mailed, and tried to stay busy.

Finally, he packed up his work, his journal, a lunch, and his guitar, and headed to the shores of Lake Washington for relief.

But there was no respite. He could think of nothing else.

> It is difficult to believe how much pain there is in the world at this moment as I look out at this placid view of the lake and mountains and life tries its best to continue around us.
>
> Everything that mattered before it doesn't matter to me anymore. I look out on these boats on the water and couldn't care less about the boats. This is all so much to bear, more than one would think the human heart could handle.

That night he and his roommates decided to turn off the TV and watch movies.

> It was the first brief escape. I am someone who can't keep one thought in my mind for more than ten seconds, and for three

days now this event has been one pro-
longed thought not only in my mind, not
only in the consciousness of the people of
the United States, but of the universal consciousness of the people of the world.

THE AFTERMATH

Tim found it was especially difficult to be so far away from
those he loved. He felt alone out West. He had just left New
York, and his friends were grieving together back there.

"The first week after the tragedy was one of the most miser-
ably lonely weeks of my life. I lost two friends, Sean and my
friend Peter. I was lucky, however. My friend Mike, who is 35,
lost four people from his wedding party. He went to four fu-
nerals in one weekend. They were all from Cantor-Fitzgerald."

Tim began to see his father, a World War II vet, with new eyes.

I now understand my father better. He is a
man of duty and a man of honor.

He kept thinking about his City, a city that was hurting.

Happy images of the time in New York fill
my mind; they are cluttered with images
from the television.

He went through a whole range of emotions. Writing
helped him acknowledge the contradictions, and sort them
through.

At first, the thoughts were confused, filled with questions.

Can we beat a country or culture that does not value life? This is bigger than anything else before us, a defining moment in our history, a new battle field, a new enemy.

There is so much information now about religion, about Christianity vs. Islam; East vs. West, who is right? Is Allah a false god, or are Allah and God the same thing?

The questions were unanswered, his thoughts disconnected.

Is this the moment where capitalism falls, is this the moment where Rome falls? What brought Rome down, was it hedonism? Who was right?

"At this point, I was angry."

We have to show them a lesson. They cannot win. We cannot give in to the evil. We have to wipe them off the face of the earth.

He was also scared.

What if they, the Arabs, already have nuclear-weapons in this country? This could be their master plan, that we become another Israel.

"I thought the world was going to come to an end. I was convinced that they had people set up *every*where. You know. I wondered, Are we going to throw a nuke there now, and then will we wind up nuking each other?"

One night he had a complete panic attack.

"I wasn't even conscious of what I was saying; all this psychobabble was coming out of my mouth."

His roommate Jessica calmed him down.

"'Tim. Nothing is going to happen to you, you're okay.' She kept saying, 'You are here with us, you're okay. Nothing is going to happen.' It was like a slap in the face. Oh my God. What the hell was I just saying?"

> But I did get scared and then I realized that
> that is what they are trying to do and that's
> letting them win.

AT SEATTLE CENTER

On Friday, there was a gathering at Seattle Center, in the shadow of the Space Needle, and Tim went there to be with people.

> People from all walks of life, all races and all
> faiths. Decorated veterans walk around in
> disbelief. Kids in their soccer uniforms
> holding their moms' hands. Large men in
> Harley Davidson uniforms. A man wearing
> a John 3:16 shirt. Another walks around
> and lights every candle that would blow out
> in the wind.

It was somber; there was a pounding of drums, but no talking. The fountain was filled with flowers. Tim sat on the grass, and opened his journal.

Seattle Center has turned into a memorial for those deceased, and for the death that has occurred in our hearts. It's hard to believe just two weeks ago this place rocked with the largest music festival in the country. Now, hardly anybody says a word as they follow the floral spiral down toward the fountain.

Candles are burning, flowers are everywhere. It smells like a funeral home here. Everyone is walking around in a daze and the place is void of smiles.

I wish I could write something to take away everyone's pain or to temporarily make them feel better.

Overcome with emotion, he could not continue. Lacking the presence of mind to compose his own words, he found comfort in what others had written.

"People had written messages in chalk, one such read simply, Trust in God. People were writing their thoughts on stickems and putting them all over.

"They left poems and post-its and notebook pages and E-mails and pictures of friends lost."

So he copied the notes that were there, the cries of others.

Love is stronger than hate

Peace.

Hell hath no fury like a nation scorned.

love the U.S.

face the storm

The placards that really got him were the notes in children's handwriting,

May God unite this country under the banner of love, freedom, and justice.

Don't lose hope, be strong and something will be good.

"The hardest to bear was the children. Children were crying, and asking innocent questions, for which there were no answers. I couldn't help but wonder, Will they grow up in fear?"

Tim didn't want to leave. There were scenes he did not ever want to forget.

"A man with two kids walked up to a firefighter and began to talk with him and thanked him. One person made murals; another assembled an American flag from flower petals, with teacup candles as the stars. Candles placed around the sides of the fountain dripped down the walls like tears."

Everyone recorded it in his or her own way.

"Some, such as me, buried their heads pensively in a notebook. Others took pictures or videos, others stared and said nothing, just trying to imprint the images in their minds."

Still at a loss for words, in the upper margin of the page, Tim drew a picture of a rosary, like a string of worry beads, a kind of prayer wheel. Fifty dots linked together for the Hail Mary's, interspersed by four bigger beads for the Our Father's and the Glory Be's; a cross where the lines came together.

"I crossed off where I was at as I said each decade."

I cannot abandon my faith, especially at such a trying moment in human history. But I cannot help but feel abandoned by God in the face of such catastrophic pain, terror and evil.

Tonight I pray for world peace, and a resolve to this horrific conflict.

PHILOSOPHICAL REFLECTIONS

Over the next few days, Tim pulled out his notebook again and again. The more he wrote, the more philosophical he became, trying to make sense out of the senseless.

Positive thought is light, and light always conquers darkness. Think good thoughts, feed yourself well. Do the things you need to do to make yourself feel better.

If we celebrate our lives with love, hate cannot conquer us. Fill your hearts with love, love for each other, a love for our great country, and love for freedom. Love is life, hate is death. If we can hold on to love, and all that is good, we can never be destroyed.

"Maybe the message is to start doing things that please you . . ."

He stops, looks off into the distance for a moment, takes a moment to compose himself, and then continues.

"Too many people are locked up in jobs that they hate, and they are miserable."

He felt a surge of patriotism.

Now is our time to show the world that we are the strongest country in the world, not just because of our economics, our military, our technology, but because we stand for freedom, and we are as strong as we are because we are the strongest spiritual country in the world. It is the spirit of America that has created the greatest nation ever, and it is this spirit of America that will allow us to prevail.

Good happens from everything. This barbaric act united the world.

God said if there were a few good people, he would spare all for these few good people. If this tragedy, this act of terrorism, has shown us anything, it is that there are a lot of good people out there.

God is love, and never before in my twenty-seven years have I seen such an outpouring of love, concern, and selflessness for my fellow Americans. The world mourns as one with us.

Perhaps this will be the trigger to a universal spirituality and a new millennium of peace.

AT GROUND ZERO

At Christmas, Tim flew back home to see his family, and went to Ground Zero.

Actually standing there stunned him; he admits that he cried in one or two places.

"I walked around the whole site. It was empty, like nothing; nothing registering, complete disbelief. It was hard to see—it is so enormous, it's mind-blowing. There is a fence around the whole area, and one part where you can walk up on a grandstand. Families were gathering there to look at it. I got to go up there.

"There was still twisted, charred, humungous heaps of metal everywhere, and drapes over a lot of the buildings. Some of the tops of the buildings were burned and charred. There are still ribbons and flowers all around it; people still bring them."

Being at the site brought a flood of memories.

"My father worked on Wall Street. When I was a little kid, on Christmas Eve, I would go into the office with him. We would take the PATH train from New Jersey to the World Trade Center and then walk to Wall Street from there.

"He took me to the top once—I was young, seven or eight years old. My overall impression was of a magnanimous, endless view. I was afraid to go near the glass railing; people were leaning over it, but I was afraid to go near it."

During his December visit, Tim stayed with his friend Tommy.

"Tommy lives in one of the most beautiful apartments in Hoboken, New Jersey, facing lower Manhattan. The room where I slept every night has a window the size of three storefront windows. It looked right out on where the WTC *was*.

"Every night there was a glow where they were working. It was like a football stadium, they have so many people working and so many lights down there. And I slept with that view every night."

Tim recalls an eerie conversation he had had in June with his friend Frost, the one who ran across the Brooklyn Bridge covered in gray dust.

"Frost and I were walking down around Battery Park looking up at the World Trade Center. Thinking about the bomb in 1993, I asked him, 'Can you believe someone tried to take those towers down? What would happen if they came down? It would take years to clean up. . . . How would New York ever recover?'"

Now he shakes his head sadly.

"Who knew?"

WHY WRITE?

Even though he couldn't bring himself to write immediately, for Tim, writing was the natural salve to turn to.

"It was just so, it was just so, it was just so shocking, and the only thing I knew to do that was still familiar and comfortable was to write.

"I don't know why the hell we write. Maybe it's innate, or maybe over the years, since I like to journal, I have conditioned myself to process things through writing."

> I can build, manipulate, structure, order and create the ideas that fill my notebooks. My world is in these pages; I am the master of it, and I control it. I can't control my feelings, but I can create order within the blue lines of my Mead notebooks.

Through writing, he talked himself through the confusion of what was happening.

"Sometimes I wrote ten, twelve, fifteen pages, while crying. I would get it all out, and the next day, I would wake up, and it was like I'd been baptized. All that stuff I was going through, wiped out."

One night, a week after September 11th, Ben's sister came over.

"I told her, 'I'm sorry I'm such a buzz kill tonight. I am so miserable, I don't want to be around people right now. I would rather stay home, and write in my journal and play my guitar and work on my screenplay.'

"They went out, and she came home early by herself, and I was a completely, completely different person. I was joking around and laughing. I don't know what I did. I guess by writing, I got something out."

Ten years ago, when Tim first started journaling, he wrote almost every night.

> My world was much smaller then. It consisted of my family, some friends, a red Volvo, the distance the Volvo covered from my home to St. Joseph's High School, high school, the girls I liked who did not like me, and soccer.
>
> It was a small world, full of the heavy thoughts of an overly analytical, overly sensitive, ambitious adolescent. Now that world is changed considerably. From that time of innocence, I went out in the world to find my way.
>
> I found love and I found out what heartbreak is. Heartbreak is something I still haven't gotten over. Heartbreak is something I am not sure you ever get over.

Tim realizes that for him, and for most people, after September 11th, life can no longer be simple.

> As the world became larger, a week ago, it became smaller, when the planes crashed into the World Trade Center and the Pentagon. Every time I begin to laugh or have a good time, the images revisit me, and the suffering of others brings a weight of sadness on my heart that is almost unbearable.
>
> The world stands poised and anxious right now. We stand and wait for what we do not know.

Heartbreak is something I am not sure you ever get over.

APPLY THIS

After the World Trade Center and Pentagon attacks, there was a sudden surge of fondness for "comfort foods": meat loaf, macaroni and cheese, apple pie, and brownies.

When the world seems dark and confusing, writing, too, is familiar and comforting. You learned to write in the first grade, maybe even earlier. There is a sense of safety in going back to what is known, and to that which is connected with the less complicated time of childhood. The ability to put your thoughts on paper is yours, and nobody can ever take that away from you.

❧ CHAPTER 7 ❧

Where Do I Go from Here?

Writing Through
to Resolution

In *Write It Down, Make It Happen*, I describe a technique I call Writing Through to Resolution. The prescription is to write out your confusion and doubt, plough through the angst and indecision, and keep on writing—you write your way right into a solution. It is a process that works, but it can use up lots of ink, and many pages of paper.

Recently my friend Patti resolved a complex problem by writing a single sentence. She posed her dilemma in writing, and let the solution take care of itself. Twenty-five words is all it took.

Patti is a registered nurse with over 30 years of hospital experience. Five years ago, she started teaching nursing at a school connected to a community hospital. The students take classes and also have clinical hours where, under supervision, they are assigned to monitor and care for patients.

Patti's approach to teaching says a lot about her nursing style: She is soft, and strict. Her passion for her work comes out in her caring—and in her insistence on accountability.

"I give my pupils freedom to be students, but I have high standards. I am easy-going as long as they work hard and work with me."

Patti has firm expectations about attendance.

"It's more than attendance; they are showing up at the hospital to do caseloads. Students know what the rules are, both in my requirements and in the objectives they need to fulfill to pass the quarter."

If a student is going to be absent, Patti insists that he or she notify her in advance. Students have her home phone number, her pager, her cell phone, and free range to call her day or night.

"If they know by 5:30 in the morning that they are not coming in, I count on being called. They are told this the first day: if they don't make it to clinical, they'd better be sick enough to have to go to the doctor. If they miss more than two clinical days, they're done. We've only got ten weeks."

So the regulations are clear: and not only do they call her, they call the unit where they are working, because everything Patti asks of her students relates back to the professional world.

"I tell them, 'I'm not trying to make you do extra work because I'm mean. I ask you to do this because there is a rational reason for it. I want to be able to look up at you from a bed one day and go, 'Oh, thank God, I trained you.'"

"NO SHOW"

Since the rules are spelled out so stringently, Patti was surprised one day recently when Tammy, one of her nursing students, did not show up, and did not call. Patti had to scramble and double up the others in order to take care of Tammy's patients.

Patti set about her morning's work. She did her rounds with her other students, she did her paperwork, got her coffee, sat down to prepare her reports: an hour into the shift and she still did not know where Tammy was, and why she hadn't called.

"That first hour is a critical hour because they have already gotten the night shift's report, they have already done all their first assessment of the patient."

Now Patti began to worry.

"It so rarely happens that a student wouldn't call, I'm thinking she got into a car crash on the freeway. So I'm fretting."

At last, Tammy called to say she wasn't coming.

Initially, Patti was relieved that the student wasn't dead or in an accident. Then she asked, "Where are you?"

Tammy replied that she had been out late the night before, and then stayed over at her boyfriend's.

Patti expressed dismay at this cavalier confession.

"And then came the attitude, and all the excuses. I was not interested in excuses. She did not come, that's all that mattered.

"I was aghast at her irresponsibility. I was so furious, I had to pace. I am rarely that angry. Her conduct disturbed me tremendously and I didn't know why."

Patti went around the rest of her day, but she couldn't stop thinking about Tammy's disregard for the rules, her arrogance and apparent indifference.

"I was trying to function and do all the work I have to do, and the whole time my head's churning. A speeded-up voice inside me is saying, 'Just relax, just relax, let it go, you're fine, you'll work it out.' I stewed on it all day, but I could not come to any answer."

DOUBT ABOUT HER TEACHING STYLE

Patti wondered if the student's laxity was indirectly her fault. Maybe she had been too lenient and easy-going with the class, and conveyed the wrong message to them.

"It disturbed me: I could just write Tammy off as someone irreverent, without common decency, without courtesy or respect for the profession, but maybe I had communicated to her that that casualness was okay."

In graduate school, Patti had studied optimum environments for studying, and for retaining information. She learned that anxiety limits not only our ability to take in new material but the capacity to access knowledge we already have.

"I like to give my students a climate free of anxiety to learn in. When they abuse my willingness to work with them, to give them leeway, I feel wounded that they could be so disrespectful of my trust and my niceness. I take it personally."

UNCOVERING THE
ROOT OF THE PROBLEM

But there was something more, and Patti knew that if she wanted to come up with a punishment that would make a difference, she had to first figure out in her own mind what that nagging concern was.

"I have learned over the years that resolution is not so much searching for the solution, but identifying the problem. That's where the work has to be. All the rest is spastic twitching, it's so un-useful."

If you want to resolve an issue, you need to understand the crux of it, what is causing the conduct in the first place.

Says Patti, "When you give a child a swat to cease bad behavior, he doesn't learn anything, he just stops the activity."

True, there may be times in conflict when you just want the activity to stop, but if your goal is a resolution that is integral and long-lasting, you need to find why there is a problem in the first place. And then let the discipline fit the offense. The best lessons come from creating a correction that addresses not the surface behavior but the motivation beneath it. In a brilliant parenting move, for example, Prince Charles took young Harry to a rehab center when he was caught drinking and smoking marijuana: not for treatment, but to see the effect drugs and alcohol could have.

Once you name the underlying concern, then the solution part falls into place; it becomes merely a matter of establishing what outcomes you want to have.

Patti still had not come to terms with what precisely about the whole thing bothered her; why was she so angry? If she knew that, she would have a clue to the elementary issue, which would point in the direction of a remedy.

It wasn't until that night when Patti sat down to write an E-mail to one of her nurse colleagues that the answer came pouring out.

We try so hard to teach them more than just
skills, as we know nursing is so much more
than that. This girl doesn't get that. She has
all the attributes to do extremely well. It
angers me that she is probably going to pass
the course, and she doesn't get it.

By writing to her friend, Patti was finally putting her finger
on what infuriated her about the student's action and attitude.

"I could teach nursing to a 15-year-old, and they probably
could do it, but nursing is not simply about proficiency. It's that
critical thinking component, the compassion, and the ability to
recognize that this is important, God-calling work that we do.
This is not a job that you can pick up somewhere; it is a vocation.

"I am at risk every day, with twenty patients and ten students. The students are taking human lives in their hands, and
my butt is on the line. I don't take that lightly, and the fact that
Tammy did was an affront to me. I was astounded that she
would think her careless attitude and selfishness were okay in
terms of this profession."

Now the question was, What to do about it? Any consequences Patti established would have to address not the absence
but the attitude. How to design a disciplinary measure to teach
the bigger lesson?

Patti discussed the dilemma with her husband.

"He's my pillar—but his style of listening is that he wants
to 'fix it,' and I didn't want him to solve it for me. I just needed
someone to listen while I worked it through."

Writing provides just that kind of attentive, non-judgmental,
non-advice-giving ear. Writing trusts you to come up with your
own plan.

PM WRITING

Patti keeps a notebook by her bedside. She often uses the technique described in the Introduction, what I call Twilight Writing—that is, recording your thoughts just before drifting off to sleep, or when first awakening, before getting up. Patti fell into bed exhausted, but before dozing off, she scribbled the burning question in her notebook:

> How can I best reprimand my student for her irresponsible behavior in a way that will not only be meaningful and appropriate, but also pivotal!

When Patti woke up the next morning, what came to her was not an answer, but a feeling of tranquility. She felt peaceful. That calm came from knowing that the answer was there, waiting for her. By consigning her quandary to the page, she now felt free to focus on whatever else she needed to do.

"I didn't have a clue how I would appeal to her, or what I would say, I just knew I had asked for help and somehow it would work."

All Patti had was her *intent* that what she came up with would matter and be right.

"I have had discussions with my children where I thought, Please God, let my words be right, because I know they will reflect on this lecture when they are older. It felt like that. Whatever I said to Tammy, I wanted it to be earthshaking, something she would remember.

"It's not that I saw myself as a great orator imparting eternal wisdom, but it was important that somehow what I said would make a difference. Tammy could choose to be the kind of nurse she could become, that it was our calling to become—or, if this wasn't her profession, she would know it and quit."

A PRETEND SCENARIO

They met in an empty patient room. Patti sat on the window ledge and her student sat on the corner of the bed.

At first, Tammy was defensive, with that same belligerence that got her into trouble in the first place.

Patti met her fierceness with a no-nonsense reply.

"The attitude has got to go. I'm here to tell you that unless it changes, you failed. So we can be done right now, or we can try to work this out, but there will be consequences. You will be required to do something and there is no negotiation."

Tammy was surprised. Her whole body language shifted. Patti softened.

"'There is something else in your life, that has gone on or is going on, someone who built a big block of wood on your shoulder, and the human, nurturing nurse part of me wants you to know I care about that.'"

But there was something else she wanted her to know.

"As a professional nurse out there being on the receiving end of your not coming in, I don't give a DAMN what your problem is, I want you in here with no excuses and I want you doing a professional day's work."

Patti later said she didn't know where the words were coming from, but she knew she would have to make it personal to reach her, to crack her veneer. She asked Tammy whom she loved most in the world, and when Tammy said her son, Patti asked her to imagine that little boy as a patient in this hospital.

"What if your son had leukemia, and the specialized nurse assigned to him got drunk the night before, and forgot to call, and the new nurse assigned to him at the last minute didn't realize that with leukemia a slight temp increase could indicate an infection that could take that young boy's life?"

By the time his nurse sobered up and called in, that little boy's life could have been irrevocably affected.

Patti told Tammy to treat any patient like her son, or like her mother, her sister—anyone she loved. How would you want them to be cared for?

"If you are assigned to nurse a child who is sick, that little boy's mother doesn't care what your life problems are, that little boy doesn't care what your problems are, and your supervisor doesn't care. Your colleague who is your good friend may care. And that's good. You need to have friends. But you also need to figure out here and now that if you are called to this profession, it is a life quest, not a day's work and a day's pay, and if you can't do it, leave."

FOLLOWING A MODEL NURSE

Patti was still not sure if she was getting through to Tammy. She replayed in her mind the question she had written out the night before: How can I best reprimand this student for her irresponsible behavior in a way that will not only be meaningful and appropriate, but also pivotal?

Just then, a nurse manager named Deborah, a woman whom Patti admired, walked by in the hall.

"That's when it came to me what I needed to do."

Patti's goal was for Tammy to know directly how selfish behavior filters down to the patient.

"I wanted her to see, and feel that, firsthand. I wanted her to understand what happens when a nurse doesn't come in, doesn't prepare, and doesn't plan."

Who better than Deborah could embody that lesson for Tammy? The modern nurse manager puts out fires all day long, caused by needing to keep the staff happy, and also having to deal with management: budget cutting, time constraints, insurance procedures, nursing shortages. Nurses are able to give less at a time when the consumer is educated and expects more.

Patti thought, "If I could have Tammy follow Deborah around for a day, it would be an education for her; maybe an epiphany."

Tammy agreed to do it and learned an important lesson from it.

WHY WRITE?

When you are trying to solve a problem, writing listens, and does not interrupt you, or barrel on with ready-made answers. In addition, writing gets at the cause underlying the effect.

"This incident was so disturbing to me, all I knew was I needed help. And I thought, 'Henriette said, Ask for help in writing and out of thin air, it will come.'

"The information was there, I knew it. Getting older has taught me to be patient. I need to ponder it for awhile, let it gel. I will come to the right conclusion in time, but sometimes retrieval is difficult. Writing helps me retrieve it quicker.

"Writing is my main tool in problem solving."

When this incident first happened, Patti felt agitated and helpless. Writing that single sentence gave her serenity, and ultimately the direction she was looking for. It clarified her intent.

"Even though I didn't know in the morning, I felt it would come to me, that when the time came, I would know what to say, when the answer presented itself, I would recognize it. And I knew it would be deep and right."

What could have been a tense and confrontational session was powerful. A defiant student walked into that conference, and a thoughtful one walked out.

"Moreover, instead of feeling upset, I felt powerful."

The assignment had its desired effect. Even as Patti had expected, spending a day with Deborah was an eye-opener for Tammy. At the end of the quarter, when she had to write up her experience, Tammy used the word Patti had hoped for to describe the change that had transpired. She said following Deborah around for the day and seeing the effect of absence on morale and ensuing scheduling complications had been an eye-opener. She called it "an epiphany."

APPLY THIS

Before going to bed at night, write out something you are grappling with, and sleep on it. Pose the problem as a question, and don't be frantic about not knowing the answer. Let the question seep into your consciousness. Your journal or notebook will listen without jumping to a conclusion. Your page will sit with the unanswered question while you get some sleep.

First thing in the morning, write up whatever comes to mind. Do not be concerned if no immediate solution is there.

Now that it is on paper, your brain is working on it.

You will be alert to the answer when it presents itself during your day.

❧ CHAPTER 8 ❧

Years After

Healing from Rape

"She said, 'Would you try going home and writing about this incident?' I said I'd think about it. She also says things like, 'If you're depressed, try to think positive.' How, I asked her, am I supposed to think positive when you are asking me to write about the most negative experience I've ever had? She said, 'You have secrets. Sometimes it's good to get them out.'"

My friend Cassie is explaining to me why she decided, at the age of 42, to write about something that happened to her when she was 19.

Cassie and I have been friends for many years, going back to our schooldays, and yet I never knew this story. She shared it with me when she heard I was writing a book about healing. We met downtown after work in a park that runs alongside the water. We went along the bike path, walking and talking, and then sat on a bench looking out at the bay.

"If this is an application of writing and healing, I can recommend it," she said.

Her insight is backed up by experts such as psychotherapist Kathleen Adams, MA, LPC, founder of the Center for Journal Therapy in Colorado and author of *The Way of the Journal*. Adams states that there are certain "therapeutic tasks for recovery from sexual abuse," which include four prongs: "to explore feelings, mourn violation, gather strength, and celebrate healing." Without specifically setting out to, Cassie covered each of these assignments in her writing.

Cassie is clever and full of life, with a great sense of humor. She has many friends and is good at her job; she is successful and happy. Only one thing is missing: She is a single woman and would like to be married.

"After yet another try with yet another man who turned out to just want to be 'friends,' I decided it was time to take a serious look at what *I* was doing to encourage this sort of non-suitor. If there was something I could do to discourage it, I was game. I'd like to have a real lasting love affair before I die instead of a fling."

Cassie wondered if the lack of a long-term relationship in her life was linked in any way to the brutal fact that as a teenager, she had been kidnapped and raped. At the advice of a friend, she went to see a counselor to try to work this out. The therapist first gave her a book about crime victims to read.

"I liked the book a lot. But the second visit, she hit the jackpot. She told me to write my story."

Cassie procrastinated for a week before she started writing. Finally even the weather seemed to be calling her to complete this unfinished business.

It feels weird to be revisiting this tale. So much has happened since then. Good things bad things—the sky is darkening now—it's actually raining. The reason I am telling this story is that maybe somewhere in it is a clue to why I don't have a man. Otherwise it seems kind of trivial to hark back to it. People seem to think it's important and needs to be talked about. I want a man, I want a lifelong companion who loves me and whom I love back. What is the reason I don't have one? Is it connected to some emotional short-circuiting that happened twenty-three years ago? I don't know, but I am willing to explore it. The rain is pouring—it's kind of a mournful summer so maybe it's the right time.

Adams notes the importance, before writing, of "creating an environment that feels safe, comfortable and nurturing." Cassie did this instinctively; she turned on the stereo, and sat in her living room at the computer, typing up this memory. The music and the Macintosh provided an emotional separation that she welcomed.

It's funny typing this. I think if I were writing it by hand it'd be different. But I'm typing it on a word processor, which gives me a little distance from the scene. So I write a sentence and stop and objectively fix the spelling or change a word. For example, I spelled a word wrong in the last sentence of the last paragraph, so I had to push the back spacer, delete the incorrect letters and type in the correct ones. So I'm telling this heavy story but I stop to edit. It's an interesting process.

I'm also listening to music. It is a so far fabulous Gary Burton CD I borrowed from my brother. The vibes are great. Bob James is on the piano and he's unrecognizable from some of the schlock he plays on his own albums. The melodies are beautiful.

So I'm writing this heavy stuff and I'm also stopping to think, God, this song is beautiful—the piano is terrific.

All these years later, it felt surprisingly soothing to write about this event—correcting spelling, listening to music and the rain outside.

"You know, I have thought about this, and wanted to write about it, for twenty years. It is my story. It's the single most important thing that's ever happened to me in my life. I have begun to write it as a narrative many times. I started writing it not long after it happened.

"'I was raped' was the first sentence. I wrote a page or two and never finished it. Where are those two pages? They are in some notebook or other, I bet."

What brought the project to a standstill was her judgment that the style wasn't right.

"I was being glib. I knew one couldn't be glib about this. It had to be a story that would show everyone what it was like that night and how awful it was and how dark. If I wrote it right, it would make me famous, it would be a feminist tract, men would be blown away, women would say, yes, that's how it is. I wanted to set the atmosphere just right, make it the story of a young girl's initiation into the world of sex. A rite of passage inflicted on a girl by men. It would not be a horror story but it would be very serious. Very gray, very dark. Even now I have an image of this piece. I sometimes feel that this story is what I have to offer the world."

She gave up on completing it. Getting it right was just too hard.

"The idea of sitting around concentrating on capturing the correct sober style is one of those discipline problems I've got. With E. B. White as a writer's role model, what chance does a girl have? I am talked out of writing before the first sentence is down—well, the second, because the first is already down: 'I was raped.'"

THE DATE

The first step in healing from rape is telling the incident exactly as it occurred. For Cassie, the evening started out as a casual date; a guy from school named John offered to take her to a party on his motorcycle, and that sounded like an interesting way to spend a Friday night. She didn't know too much about John except that he had a crush on her friend Molly, but then, every guy in the known world had a crush on Molly.

As the words poured out of her onto the page, Cassie was astonished at the particulars that came to mind two decades later, down to the cut of John's hair, and what she had on.

> I actually even remember what I was wearing that day—or at least my memory thinks I do. I was dressed in a very pretty two-piece

suit, a mini skirt and a jacket. The jacket was fitting so it was very flattering and I felt pretty every time I put this suit on. Sheer panty hose and sling backs. And a pocket-book. I always carried a stylish shoulder bag in those days. That day, I stashed a little pinky ring in my bag—it was a gift from Molly, who was my best friend. I wore it all the time. A little silver band is all it was but it was worth a lot to me. This day it must have been bothering my finger because I took it off. I never took it off, but this night I did. It had something to do with the motorcycle.

The party was quite a few miles away, and when they got there, John started drinking and then went downstairs into the basement and got high smoking pot with some Hispanic girls who didn't speak English.

John's friend, who had a car, offered to take them home. John got into the back seat with one of the Spanish-speaking girls and Cassie was in the front with John's friend. Before long, it became awkwardly apparent what was going on in the back seat, and the driver turned to Cassie and suggested leeringly that he and she do the same. When she refused, he put her out of the car. In the middle of the night, in the middle of a strange neighborhood.

Dr. Miriam Kalman Harris, editor of the collection *Rape, Incest, Battery: Women Writing Out the Pain*, speaks of the transcendence of the "writing cure" as a procedure "moving a violent event . . . from inner to outer and then to inner again." Part of this process entails "remembering, connecting, owning." Cassie writes,

It was a dark night. It all happened in the dark. I sleep now with a light on. Probably related.

She walked the unlit streets in her little tan suit and slingbacks with her handbag, looking for a phone booth or a fire station, hoping for a taxi, when a car drove by. The car slowed down, backed up and began to cruise menacingly beside her, the men in it heckling her out the window. She crossed the street to get away from them; they circled back. Before she could even register what was happening, the car stopped, and one of the men jumped out with a knife and forced her into the back seat.

Funny little points came back to her now—the side of the street she was walking on when he grabbed her, how his rough hand felt on her mouth. And she distinctly recalls her psychological state:

> There was no escape. I was in a car. No use screaming. No use doing anything. I couldn't believe it. That is, it seemed unreal. I remember this clearly: An almost visible curtain went down in my mind. I closed myself off from what was about to happen. I left one reality behind and entered this one. But I didn't want this one to taint that one, so I closed a curtain on it. It was almost a physical feeling, this curtain coming down. We were carrying on this polite conversation as if I weren't someone they'd just kidnapped. I went along with it. The curtain was down.

Ruth Peachey, MD, a consultant in Research and Social Psychiatry, explains this extraordinary survival technique of detachment.

"Numbing out is a way of dealing with what is intolerable, of defending against and enduring severe abuse without losing one's sanity. Technically, it is called 'disassociation.'"

Disassociation means you are psychologically leaving your body. You are up here, looking down, watching what is happening.

Cassie continued, "You'd have thought we were buddies at the pool hall if you'd listened. But I didn't say anything that was true so I guess they didn't either."

They took her to an abandoned building and all pretend niceness was off; they threw her to the floor and raped her repeatedly.

I remember at one point thinking, "Oh God, I can't wait until Monday. I can't wait until this is over and I'm back being bored in school. Oh God, I can't wait to be bored again. Oh, just to be bored again."

Kathleen Adams points to the clarification and catharsis of getting it down on paper.

"Writing about memories of abuse allows [the survivor] to define her or his own reality, perhaps for the first time, without minimization or distortion."

As the details of that nightmare night filled page after page, Cassie told the facts straight, and as she did so a gradual dawning came over her.

I am writing things that I have never told anyone in my entire life. When I see them in script I think, "Well, geez, that's not so bad—you can live with that."

It is hard for Cassie to understand the kind of people who would hurt a young girl.

> It's unbelievable to me that people treat each other so poorly. I mean, you yell at your friends, you resent your parents, you don't do a favor for someone when you might have. But being really cruel—some part of their souls is dead and it makes them worthless people. The world would have been better off if they'd never been born.

At the time, she felt singled out, like these guys were out looking for her.

> But in fact they just were random predators among many. The rest of them are out there doing the same damn thing to a million other girls and women who are just trying to get home. The world is full of these jerks and they all think it's just fine and proper to treat people this way.

The men continued to abuse her and hurt her. When she passed out from the terror and the pain, they left her for dead.

The rest is a blur. Somehow she got to a hospital, and gave the police a report, but nothing ever came of it.

ANGER AT JOHN

Typing her story helped Cassie to face her feelings of anger at John and his friend, feelings she had repressed. The intensity of her emotion surprised her. It felt good to get it out.

Where is John now? Did he turn out to be a nice man with children or did some hoodlum knife him for being a punk? Is he still just a wise guy or is he a dad who's giving his kids a hard time for being like he was? I can't picture him today.

Whatever became of that other guy, John's friend, the driver who put me out on the street? I kind of hope he's dead, but if he isn't, I'd like to see him again and tell him what happened that night. I'd like to look up John the next time I'm home. I'd like to look him up in his college alumni book and tell him what happened to a young girl on a Friday night because of him. Maybe he's dead already. Maybe he got killed in Vietnam. It's a weird world. Maybe the other guy got killed in Vietnam—that'd be fine with me. He was a cold-hearted bastard and probably always would be no matter what. John was just a bastard. I'd like to yell at both of them. They were stupid stupid boys. Maybe John got AIDS. I bet he at least ended up with herpes.

And, looking back, she experienced again what finally triggered the tears.

> The first time I let myself cry was when I looked in my shoulder bag and discovered that in addition to taking my money, they'd stolen the little silver pinky ring from Molly. What could they possibly have gotten for that, a ring that was worth worlds to me? I hated them at that moment. That was when I cried and cried and cried.

Cassie came to another realization as she typed. She was alive in the fullest sense of that word. And her delight in her own vitality is Adams's third and fourth therapeutic tasks, mentioned above: to "gather strength, and celebrate healing." As Harris puts it, "Writing functions not only as a catharsis of the soul but as a record of the heroic enterprise of regaining self-power."

> Those guys are in their 50s or 60s now. The police charges were kidnap, assault, robbery, and rape. They have probably both been in jail or even murdered in a drunken brawl. That's the lives they got. I don't know why they had to grow up half human with only half the heart and soul some of the rest of us got. That was a bum break for them. I'm glad I got the deal I got and even though I think those guys should have known better than to treat me so shitty, I'm sorry their

lives were so dismal and meaningless that
they thought rape would be fun.
I am alive, hallelujah.

And Cassie is glad that she wrote it out.

"I would encourage anyone who is holding back a secret like this to type it up.

"Now that it's on paper, it doesn't seem to matter as much."

Approaching it like homework made it easier. She let go of obsessing about form and got to the core of it.

"This assignment made it possible to write about it without worrying about style and E. B. White's approval. It was like writing a letter. Like being back in college, hammering away every day on the typewriter. Very freeing. Plus it felt worthwhile.

"Typing the truth is a worthwhile activity."

APPLY THIS

There is a freedom and release that comes from consigning what has been bottled up for years to scraps of paper. Put on some music. Whatever your story is, tell the incident exactly as it occurred. Explore your feelings, gather your strength, and celebrate your wholeness.

CHAPTER 9

Interview with a Critical Mother

Listening to Her Own Body

It's known as PTSD, post-traumatic stress disorder, and we know now that it is not just experienced by war combatants who are shell-shocked. Victoria had a physical response to writing about her mom when she participated in an activity I assigned in my writing class. The exercise taught her some important things about her past. Through it, she came to a place of peace.

We rendezvoused at Coffee Animals, a funky Capitol Hill espresso shop, surrounded by glass-blown art. I was so engrossed in her tale, I hardly noticed how noisy it was, with the banging of the portafilter, the hissing of the steaming wand, the buzz of table talk around us. Once Victoria started her story, I was mesmerized. All background din melted away.

GROWING UP

Victoria had a childhood she would just as soon forget. Her mother was an alcoholic, often irrational.

Victoria's mother figured out her husband was having an affair when she was driving downtown one day and saw him walking down the street carrying another woman's dry cleaning. She confronted him, and they got divorced. Victoria was two, her brother not even a year old.

"I never had friends over; I was afraid my mother would lose it in front of them at any time. It was not just drink. She would wake up in the morning being out of control and awful. Once when she was drunk, she pulled a knife on a woman at a party. She had a lot of anger in her. Life was a daily trauma.

"When I was going through it, I thought, This woman is crazy, but I didn't know any different. I thought, Doesn't everybody have a situation like this? I normalized something that was not normal."

Victoria had a mental trick that helped her survive.

"Every day I thought, No matter how bad this day is, I don't ever have to relive it. I don't have to think about it. It was a relief to know I would not have to experience that day again; once was enough. It was a safety mechanism. That was how I coped."

THE INTERVIEW:
I AM TALENTED / SHE IS NOT

In the class, we did an imaginary interview, a written exercise to facilitate a conversation with what I call the Critic, the nagging voice inside your head that keeps you from moving forward.

The instructions are to give your Critic a name, set up a figmental conference, and enter into a dialogue. You have my permission to talk back, maybe for the first time in your life. It is all done in writing.

Victoria, whose nickname is Vikki, was skeptical.

I encourage people to create a buffer if they like. Instead of confronting the Critic directly, which might be intimidating, I suggest creating the part of an interviewer asking questions about you in the third person. Critic and interviewer alternate question and answer. Every student in the class, except Vikki, did it that way.

What Vikki did was unusual. She had a celebrity host interrogate herself and her Critic at the same time, a three-way discourse.

"The word 'interview' made me think of Barbara Walters, a powerful person. I respect her for what she has done.

"I have to say I had no idea what I was doing. I just let my pen roll. I was astonished at what came out, right away. It didn't even feel like me writing."

> **Barbara Walters:** Vikki and I want to meet her Critic, please step forward and identify yourself. We have some questions.

"I was thinking, this is not going to happen; this is not going to work."

And then, Barbara Walters says,

> **BW:** Hello Constance.

"This astonished me because I didn't expect my mother to be there, and she hates the name, Constance. She likes to be called Connie."

The interview continues,

> I am Barbara Walters, and I would like to know more about you.

Immediately Vikki's mother introduces herself in self-congratulatory terms.

> **C:** I am an artist, and a talented one. Actually I am excellent.

Then she turns mean.

> My daughter will never be as good as I am. As a matter of fact, she has no talent. I am embarrassed by her behavior and know she will never amount to anything.

There is a slight pause. And then,

> I have made sure of that.
> **BW:** How did you do that?
> **C:** I put her down all the time. I made sure she had no confidence. I destroyed her. I made her feel like she was not capable of doing anything right.
> **BW:** It looks like Vikki's head is spinning.
> **C:** I created confusion and chaos for her growing up, and to make sure she continues the process, now I put thoughts in her head.
> **BW:** Vikki says she feels like she is choking.

C: I am strangling her. I am jealous of her. Jealous of her talents and abilities. I can see she is powerful, full of energy, positive energy that I want to choke out of her. She is nothing. I like to tell her that if only she would listen to me.

BW: Vikki, are you okay?

V: Thanks, Barbara, for asking. No, I feel like my head is about to explode, or come off my neck. My throat is tightening.

BW: It's okay, Vikki, let it out. You are a powerful, intuitive, and smart woman. Tell the inner Vikki to let it go, that you can and do and will protect her. She is safe. No one can hurt her ever again, especially her mother. Let it go. Live on, empower yourself, Vikki. God loves you. Please let it go.

Vikki, tell Constance how you feel, and then shut that door of pain and confusion. Tell her to let you go.

TALK BACK

What poured out of her pen next were the strongest and most confident words Vikki had ever conceived.

V: Mom, I love you and I need you to know it's okay for me to be happy. I want to be happy, and I am happy, and there is nothing you can do anymore to stop me. I refuse to let you control me. I have had it with your

> criticism, with your negative everything. In
> spite of you, I will succeed, and be free of
> criticism and negativity. I smile with happi-
> ness. It flows through me. I am free of pain,
> and of you. I am my own person. I am no
> longer choking. I feel better. I love myself. I
> am an artist. I am talented. I have no more
> critics, only an inner coach.

When she rereads that brave statement now, Vikki is astonished at her own forthrightness.

"The supportive atmosphere of the class made it okay to be
me, and to claim the artistic side of me."

Amazed that her daughter took so staunch a stand, the mom
on paper backed down, and even softened with the following
extraordinary concession.

> **Connie:** I am proud of you. I want you to be
> free. I have been wrong all these years to
> criticize you. I am going to encourage you
> from now on. You are right; you deserve to
> be happy, to be free of my negativity. You
> have courage, you are brave, you will light
> up the world with your creativity and bril-
> liance. You are a star and I want you to shine.

VALIDATION

Vikki felt emotionally exhausted and physically drained when
she finished. She was also amazed, for she did not expect this to
happen when she first began the exercise.

"I had never done anything like this. It sounded so bizarre. I didn't think it would work."

That night, she wrote an entry in her journal trying to assess what had taken place.

> I wrote to the Critic even though I was choking. My throat was tightening to the point of pain. I could physically feel my throat closing. It felt like someone had their hands around my neck, clamping down harder and harder. My passageway was becoming narrower and narrower. The symptoms were so intense that it didn't matter that no one was actually hurting me, it was very much real. My neck still hurts now, and that was over two and a half hours ago.
>
> It amazes me that I kept on writing. Even as my throat was closing down and it was difficult to breathe, I was still able to stay focused on the interview. Later, I couldn't believe that I continued to write, and that I was extremely calm. It never occurred to me to stop; I just kept on with the interview among Barbara Walters and Constance and me.

When Vikki came to class the next day, she shared her dialogue with others in a small group. One of the students was also a therapist. When she heard Vikki's description of her head spinning, she noted that that characteristic was a classic symptom of PTSD, post-traumatic stress disorder. She told Vikki that whenever she worked with post-traumatic stress cases, they all said the same thing: that their head was spinning.

The therapist thought it was quite probable that Vikki had been strangled as a child.

That afternoon, Vikki went to the library and looked the topic up.

"I got books on PTSD and I started reading them."

What she found corroborated what the therapist in class told her. For example, Dr. Aphrodite Matsakis, author of *I Can't Get Over It*, says "flashbacks are not a sign that you are losing your mind, but rather that some traumatic material is breaking forth into your consciousness."

In addition, Matsakis explains somatic (bodily) reexperience of trauma.

"During somatic flashbacks, a physical pain or medical condition emerges as a means of expressing the feelings and bodily states associated with trauma."

Vikki shared the interview with her husband.

"He had a look on his face of great concern. He said, 'You know, we have been together for 23 years, and ever since I have first known you, you never let me touch you around the sides, or the back of your neck without flipping out.'"

Then he reminded her of something else: she had gone a few years ago to an ear, nose, and throat specialist for allergies, and when the doctor examined her, he told her that she had a broken nose, and that it had occurred in childhood.

"Then my husband said to me softly, 'I think you're right. I think your mother strangled you.'

"I felt it in the pit of my stomach when he talked about it."

Vikki felt validated by the therapist, the texts, and her husband.

"I believe that, yes, I did get choked, although it's irrelevant at this point. As a child I was not allowed to talk. If I was in an argument with my mother, or if I disagreed, I couldn't speak.

So my experience with the interview was a symbol of my voice being silenced. The important thing was that now I felt relieved. I felt hopeful and happy."

PEACE IN HEAD

"When I was started this process, I recognized that I had a negative voice in my head all the time, but I didn't think it would be my mother. In retrospect, I realize that Barbara Walters was the perfect person. She protected me. I needed a powerful woman to defend me, one my mother would respect. I felt more comfortable with her there."

For Vikki, this exercise resolved emotional issues that were present below the surface.

"I didn't realize how much my mother was still in my head, until I sat down and did this interview. It made perfect sense when it came together. Now I understand.

"I lived in fear of her all these years—until last week. I was afraid if I said the wrong thing, I would get hurt. I don't feel that way now. I am not going to give away my power."

Years ago, her mother gave Vikki a painting she always hated. She went home and threw it out.

"I don't have fear any more; I totally let go.

"My head is so quiet. I have peace—I can sit and have nothing in my head."

THANKS, BARBARA WALTERS

There were a few points of last-minute business, and Vikki took care of them at the end of her interview.

Barbara: Thank you, Connie, for showing up. Thank you for being so honest. Vikki appreciates your letting her go. Thank you for freeing her. She needed to do that. You were great.

Vikki would like to continue a discussion with you; when would you like to talk again?

Connie: How about next Friday at 5:00?

BW: Is that okay with you, Vikki?

V: 5 pm next Friday would be great, thank you.

I am smiling. Nothing will stop me now. Thank you, Barbara Walters. Thank you, Connie. This has been one of the more intensive experiences of my life. Definitely a life-changing event.

APPLY THIS

Imagine the strength that you might feel telling off someone in your life who has put you down, made you feel small. Wrap the response of Vikki's mom around you: "I am proud of you. I want you to be free. I have been wrong all these years to criticize you. You are a star and I want you to shine." Who in your life do you need to hear similar sentiments from? Have an honest conversation in the safe presence of a mediator, a third-party who is totally nonjudgmental. Just the facts, ma'am, and the freedom to express them. Set it up as though you and the other party were both being interviewed by a famous media anchor. It's okay if the celebrity, although impartial, leans a little toward your side of the story. After all, you are the casting director of this one, and it is your show.

Notice that Vikki also followed my recommendations for ending an interview with the Critic.

1. Thank the Critic for coming.

2. Set a date and time for your next meeting.

When you make that appointment to meet again, keep that engagement as scrupulously as you would attend to an actual appearance on a famous TV talk show.

You can do this imaginary interview as many times as you like. It gets richer with repetition, and is always something you can go back to, especially when you feel stuck.

By the way, you don't have to believe it will work for it to work!

❦ CHAPTER 10 ❧

Way to Whine

Hosting Your Own Pity Party

In the 1980s, Dr. James Pennebaker of the University of Texas studied groups of college students in a pioneering experiment. His clinical research showed that students who wrote out their problems had an increase in germ-fighting lymphocytes, and paid fewer visits to the infirmary.

Leslie is a college sophomore. She comes from a small town, and is far away from home, living in a co-ed dorm. She told me she uses writing as a kind of a dumping ground, a place to get out whatever is bothering her. Dr. Pennebaker would approve.

Leslie and I met on campus in the Student Union building; she made sure we found a quiet place in a side corridor where we could have at least some element of privacy amid the collegiate bustle.

149

LETTING THE BEAST OUT

"My friends and I have a joke that in your journal you can show the ugly side of you. I was rereading my journal this morning, and it's quite funny, some of the awful things I say in here. The entries are honest and they are humorous. I was obviously in a rage at that point; overly tired or overly stressed at another point.

"I call it the ugly side because these are things I would never ever say to any of these people face-to-face. This is my own selfish person."

And it feels good to get it out.

Leslie writes out with abandon her complaints about her roommate, her "boy issues," her diatribes against her crew coach. Writing is a valve that lets off steam, a catharsis.

After, she is ready to face the world.

A CHANCE TO REBEL

Leslie hosts her own "Pity Party" when she writes. That means she indulges herself in the luxury of feeling sorry for herself, getting in a tizzy, or blowing a fuse, without hurting anyone. Her journal is a safe place to be angry. She knows she can scream and cry on paper, and she is not afraid to say whatever is on her mind. She knows it is better to have a conniption and get heated in writing than to speak out loud something she might later regret. Ferocious feelings lose some of their intensity once they are expressed in writing. Writing tames the wild beast.

> I want to rebel so badly. I don't care what
> anyone thinks. I am sick of people who get
> in my way. Don't get in my way. No more

> walking all over me. I am a raging bitch. No
> more pathetic girl.

Leslie goes on for pages, as she calls it, "ranting and raging," and then she gets over it. It passes. She feels more calm.

> I will be a dedicated, fun, feisty, laughter-
> oriented, petite woman. Dates will fly at
> me. Next quarter it will all be okay.

SEPARATING BIG
DEALS FROM LITTLE ONES

"Pity Party Writing" reduces unnecessary altercations, and raises the quality of those fights you do get into, because it gives you a chance to release the worst of it, and find out what you are really mad about.

"Writing lets me get out irrational and rational feelings all in one. Then I go back later to figure out what went on. That is why I laugh when I look at my journal now. The things I worried about are minute now, but three months ago they loomed large."

For example, Leslie fills almost a whole notebook with tirades about her roommate, Mary.

"Obviously when you live with someone, little things are going to tick you off at certain times. In one of the passages I am going off because she is making too much noise; she is rustling too much. How can you rustle too much? It is just ridiculous."

> Mary is shuffling, making noise, and it is
> pissing me off. She crackles around at night,

and in the morning she is so freakin loud. I
am tired of this!

"It is funny to look at that. I like Mary. We are friends, we
get along, but it is close quarters being roommates; you can't
help getting annoyed. So I write down,

'It is driving me nuts' . . .

and then I realize something like that is habit; and it is like complaining about how someone brushes her teeth. What's the
point in bringing that up? You can't. Is she going to change the
way she brushes her teeth? It will just end up driving her crazy.
I would rather write it down. That way it's out, over, I'm done
with it. I don't have to verbalize it."

Also, Leslie can look back on previous entries and realize
that that's not the first time she has written about Mary's clatter,
so it's a habit of hers.

"It's the way she is. She is a loud person, even in the way she
throws her books down. She doesn't mean anything by it. She
has done it all year, and I have written about it all year. So I can
say it's just one of her habits, like when someone slams the door
shut; it is nothing personal."

I am not trying to start something I am
just sick of this noise. I know she cannot
help it. She is just loud and restless in the
mornings.

"Once I write it down, I can look at my roommate and say,
So what, she makes a racket? I am sure I do things that she is

not exactly happy with either. I am sure I make too much noise sometimes, too."

Another issue was food.

> I am not rooming with Mary ever again. She purposely is trying to make me fat by buying things I like.

> Pity Party Writing puts things in perspective.

> Mary cannot define my body. Only I can.

When you write down what you are upset about, you get clear on your own underlying needs and motivations, and learn to choose your battles carefully. Writing gives you a chance to reflect on what is bothering you and decide, Is this the hill you want to die on?

"I realize what's little and what's big, what's worth fighting about and what's not worth fighting about."

SORTING OUT
THOUGHTS FROM FEELINGS

Writing is useful in sorting through thoughts and feelings, especially when it comes to "boy issues."

Leslie's entries about Steve show her frustration with him, almost from the start:

> I met this person—his name is Steve, I really like him. Why isn't he calling? Why

> am I always the one to initiate the conversa-
> tion? Or the idea to go for coffee?

She was getting mixed messages from him. He was friendly and polite, and often seemed to go out of his way to be with her. Other times, he ignored her. It was confusing.

> I am very attracted to Steve and I do not
> think he remotely likes me. Does he like me
> or want me to leave him alone, or what?

Typical of Steve was the afternoon he stood Leslie up when they were scheduled to work out together.

"I had asked him to go run with me; we jog together every week. Instead, he and a friend went down to the gym to play racquetball. I got upset and wrote about it. I thought he was making an excuse, which he probably was."

> I called Steve yesterday to ask if he wanted
> to go running. He said sure, he'd love to,
> but he went to the gym and got too sore to
> run. I was like, Yeah right, racquetball wa
> wa. He started laughing, but I got my point
> across. I am not impressed with him contin-
> uing to ditch me.

Steve was her crush, but meanwhile, right under her nose, her friend Mark was crazy about her, but at first she was not paying attention to the signals.

> I have a wonderful friend in Mark. I thank
> God for him. He allows me to be myself.

I never feel ashamed around him, and I am
comfortable with the way I am when he
is near.

Mark is kind and thoughtful.

We talked, shared a beer, and he made
me a jelly sandwich. He remembered I was
allergic to peanut butter.

He is gentle and good, and I had a great
time with him. He is much more direct to
speak to than Steve. I appreciate how easy it
is to be friends with him.

The more she wrote about Mark, the more Leslie starting
noticing his positive attributes.

Good points about him are his friendliness
and ability to make me feel beautiful, his
courage, his ability to know what is important. He and I danced at the dance. I was
too intimidated to dance with Steve.

One day, Leslie wrote two side-by-side lists contrasting the
qualities of Steve and Mark. It was simply meant as a comparison between two guys in her life. Ironically, it was not until
months later that she got what she had done.

As mentioned earlier, your writing speaks back to you, sometimes startling you with something you don't remember you said.

Now Leslie is surprised when she looks back on those two
lists. It did not sink in when she wrote, at the bottom of Steve's
column,

not sure, not sure

and, after cataloguing Mark's qualities,

I am in trouble.

"I am in trouble because I was starting to fall in love with him. I wrote that before I started dating him, and I didn't remember that I had written it."

PROCRASTINATION.
PLAIN AND SIMPLE

When you have a record of your whining, it provides an insight into destructive patterns.

"After awhile, I start to see patterns in my life; I am complaining about the same things over and over again. Even without rereading, I know when I am writing it that I have griped about this more than once. It feels familiar."

> I am so sick of being so behind in school.
> I have wasted so much of this quarter.

"Seeing that spelled out is a harsh reality check. I'm stubborn. It is hard for me to admit that I am doing things that are not healthy for me, until I see it repeated."

> This quarter I focused on all the wrong things.
> I need to catch up.

"When I see that complaint more than once, or I am conscious of writing it before, I think to myself, Well, maybe if I didn't procrastinate so much . . . "

My goal tonight is to make lists of all I have
to do. I am not going to fail out. I have come
too far in this school.

"This quarter, I am no longer journaling about being behind."

MAKING HEALTHY
CHOICES AND CHANGES

Grousing in writing motivates change. Through writing, Leslie
came to a decision about her involvement with crew. She realized how constantly she was complaining about the coach,
complaining about the team, and there are repeated notations
such as

> Only nine weeks left
> Only eight weeks left
> I can do this
> I can finish this

"I was not taking care of myself. I wasn't getting any sleep.
I wasn't getting my studies done. I wasn't eating right. A lot of
it had to do with being involved in crew. It was a lot of pres-
sure. You have to get up at 4:00 in the morning."

> I am not going to crew tomorrow. I need to
> study. My energy is tapped out and I no
> longer have excuses.
> I am so tired, baby.

> I sit here and struggle because I do not want
> to go to practice. The coach puts too much
> demand on me. I want to take off and do
> what I want to do.

When Leslie got seriously injured and could not row for three weeks, it was a revelation to her.

"I thought I owed it to people to be in a team sport, but I don't have to do the things I don't want to do."

Then another awareness hit her.

"Before my injury, every day I'd wake up, and run to rowing practice. After paddling in the lake for an hour, I'd run back to the dorm. That was my favorite part: running to and from practice. So I just cut out the rowing part. I still get up at 4:00 A.M. and run. I do what I enjoy, instead of doing what I hate, just to please other people. I don't have to please anyone but myself."

LESSON LEARNED
FROM A FAMILY CRISIS

Because Leslie is comfortable using her journal working through mundane matters, when she comes up against something huge, she can turn to writing.

"My journal was the first thing I reached for on September 11th. I sat in front of the TV with my notebook and recorded news updates. I was not ready to process my own thoughts, but I had to write."

Recently Leslie had a heartbreaking crisis at home. A close family member committed suicide. At first she was too stricken to write her feelings, but she found comfort in recording the stark facts. How she got the news. Where she was when the call came. The details of what happened. The trivia around the day that took on portentous import.

"It was the 13th of the month. I woke up that morning and wrote,

> It's going to be a full moon today. The sky looks dark. It is going to be a very unlucky day today.

"And later that day I got the call. It was shocking to look back and see that stupid superstition at the top of the page."

LIFE IS PRECIOUS— FOLLOW YOUR PASSION

"Before I didn't have a direction, and now I do."

When her relative took his life, it cemented her resolve to work with sick people.

"My mom said something after the suicide in my family: 'Life is not short, life is precious.' Why not go to school to study something you are passionate about? My passion is to nurse people who are dying. I would like to work in Trauma and ER."

And she set herself a daunting goal: to travel from one coast to the other by cycling.

> I want to be a vibrant, alive, beautiful woman. I want to live a crazy, adventurous, loving life.

I will ride my bike across the nation,
and I will do well in school. I am not scared
anymore. I want to live a long life. I am
leaving worry behind me.

And she came to a healthy resolution. She was tired of chasing Steve.

Am I not good enough for him?

She wrote him a letter of good-bye and stapled it into her journal.

Dear Steve, at one point, I wanted you in my life. You do not make time for me, and that hurts my feelings. I have made so much time for you. I found a good friend who understands that friendship is a two-way street. This guy treats me like a queen.

I cannot continue to hold on to the hope that you are going to show up in my life and try to get to know me. I am sick of longing, hoping, waiting, and hurting. You have no say over me any longer.

Leslie did not mail the letter to Steve.
"It's not anything he needs to see; it was written just for me."
And then she wrote a letter to Mark. This one she did deliver.

Dear Mark, you amaze me in the way you make me feel. I feel so good with you. I could just chill. Let's hang out more.

WHY WRITE?

James Pennebaker's study makes sense to Leslie. She sees the connection in her own life between writing and being healthy.

"Writing is a stress relief. Some students take a warm shower or exercise. I personally like journaling and long runs. I jog, and then sit, and be with my journal."

Why does it make a difference to write, rather than, say, talk over your particular problems with a friend? Leslie has several answers to that. For one thing, writing is more private.

"I am a private person. This is a small school. People are curious by nature; they want to know what is going on. They listen to what you say to another person."

A journal keeps your problems confidential. And it does not raise an eyebrow, which might make you falter, or change the subject.

"I'd rather write it down in a journal where it is just me seeing it. When I talk it out, I am not always as honest, and often don't explore the topic fully."

For another reason, the page has endless patience.

"I like to wallow in my pity. My friends will not put up with that for long. Friends can only take so much of your moaning and groaning. If they are your friends at all, they will call you on it if they are healthy people, and tell you to get off it, or go to a counselor."

A journal is a way to ramble incessantly and not have someone talk back to you or say stop.

"Eventually your own brain is going to say, I have had enough.

"That's what happened with Steve. If you notice in my journal, it just cuts off. I'm done. Move on. Here is my final letter to him. It took me many months to get to that place, but when I'm done, I'm done. I dealt with that."

Leslie is quiet for a moment, and then adds thoughtfully, a final advantage to writing.

"I give a lot of time for others; taking fifteen minutes a day to write is time for me. Fifteen minutes for me lets me be a healthier friend."

APPLY THIS

Wring your hands, gnash your teeth, pound the pillow—or seethe and vent all about it in your journal.

❦ CHAPTER 11 ❦

A Pattern of Abuse

Connecting the Dots

Debra is on the Leadership Council of Survivors in Service (SIS), an organization that brings together those who have lived through domestic violence, and now help others in a similar situation. She invited me to do a presentation on goal setting at their annual retreat, and then told me her own life history.

"I don't mind sharing my story with you. In SIS, we think it is important to talk about our experiences as normally as possible, because it takes away the pain of silence for us."

For 16 years, Debra lived with a violent husband. When she finally got the courage to say "Enough!", writing helped her keep her sanity and sort out what had happened. She used the "stream of consciousness" approach to writing, coined by psychologist William James and advocated by Julia Cameron. Debra labeled her 70-sheet Mead notebooks "Daily Dialogue," because they were a conversation with herself, and sometimes they turned into a conversation with her former spouse.

Her "Daily Dialogue" helped Debra connect the dots, letting the full picture emerge and cementing her resolve not to return to him.

"There are signs, but you don't know they are signs. You don't associate the behavior with emotional abuse, or withholding, or isolation. As I wrote, I could see the pattern, and the repetition."

FROM FASHION
COLLEGE TO SEAMAN'S WIFE

Debra grew up in Fort Pierre in a blue-collar, hard-working, traditional household, with a large extended family. She had no experience around the subject of domestic violence.

"My dad was a generous, creative, loving, stable individual and my mother the same."

Her parents supported her in her dreams. Debra went to Lucerne, Switzerland, to study at a fashion college for six months; her mom sewed at home to help her pay for it, and sent her $20 to $25 a week, to buy train tickets for trips to Paris, Rome, and Florence.

Then Debra decided to go to California, which is where she met Mike. He was in the Navy, stationed in San Diego.

"Mike was not happy in the Navy; in hindsight, twenty years later, I realize that he told me just enough to keep me hooked, to get me to care for him. He actually started his emotional assault early by lying."

When Debra found out she was pregnant with their first child, he thought he'd better tell her the truth: he was already married.

Mike started the divorce proceedings from his first wife, and Debra went with him to meet his family. While they were there, his stepdad flew into a tantrum, the likes of which she had never seen before. Debra crouched in the corner crying while the man shouted and screamed and called his 16- and 17-year old stepdaughters, Mike's sisters, vulgar names.

Instead of giving her second thoughts about the wedding, this scene confirmed what her future husband had told her about his stepdad.

"He told me he hated his stepfather. He said, 'This is what I don't want.'"

He married her the day his divorce came through, and the next day, Stephanie was born. Debra became a wife and mother within 24 hours.

REMOVED FROM HER SUPPORT SYSTEM

Getting military housing wasn't easy, so Debra and the baby went to live with her parents, and when Mike finished the last few months of his Navy tour of duty, he joined them there.

"I would say that was the beginning of the trouble. He was no longer in the Navy. In the Navy, he had been a cook, and he augmented his income doing pizza delivery. So now he became a pizza delivery driver."

Debra worked at Payless Drug Store as a checker. Her parents watched Stephanie for no charge while Debra was at work, but life on two minimum-wage salaries was difficult.

"He would start arguments. He said he wanted to move. He made me so miserable, I would have agreed to anything.

"With a six-month-old baby, you don't stop to think, 'Oh, I'll get a divorce with my Payless checker job.'"

They moved two hundred miles away from her family, uprooting her from everything that was familiar.

"In domestic violence terms, we call that isolation—effectively taking me from my support system."

Money was tight, and Mike was still not happy. Now when they had fights, he threw the furniture around. Debra started putting things like chairs, the stereo, and lamps in safer positions whenever he started yelling, to keep them from getting broken.

"He hated his job. He said the supervisor was mistreating him. He went to school, and then he quit school because it was too hard; because he couldn't get good grades, the GI Bill would not cover him.

"I was very alone, and not encouraged to make friends of my own. I couldn't take it anymore, and I went back to my family. That was the first time I ever left."

By that time, she had three children. When she got to her parents' house, she found that she was pregnant with her fourth.

"X comes knocking on the door—I call him X, not 'my ex,' just the letter X, meaning he is nothing to me. X comes knocking on the door saying, It's easy to get a job in California, and I promise I'll be good. I want this family. All the things you want to hear when you're eight months pregnant.

"I shut my eyes and followed. "

As soon as she got down there, she realized it was a mistake. It was nothing like he said it was. The economy was bad and jobs were scarce. At home, the violence was escalating.

CRYING AND CLEANING
UP THE MESS AFTER UPROAR

Food and drink were frequent triggers to upheaval and uproar. He drank a lot of beer, and then used the empty bottles as flying weapons. When he got mad during dinner, he threw first his plate and then the whole table.

"Anything would make him turn over the dining room table; you never knew when it was coming. Just upend the table, and then leave us to clean up all the food on the floor. It made the kids cry; it made us all cry."

Debra wasn't equipped to handle what was happening.

"I just remember trying hard to put things together. And I started to feel tired and worn out by all that.

"It got to the point where we were happier when he was not there."

If the children misbehaved, he slapped them and kicked them.

He called it discipline, but he was hurting them.

"He was a man who lived to have boys—he's big, 6 ft., 240 lbs. I never understood why he was even harder on the boys than on the girls."

If he did not like the way the children cleaned their rooms, he shouted at them and yelled insults, tearing their mattresses off the bed frames and throwing them on the floor, screaming, "Now you really have something to clean up!"

HER JOB WAS TO KEEP HIM HAPPY

Today Debra knows that financial control is a sign of an abusive relationship. She was in charge of the checkbook, the shopping, the bills, but he had no responsibility, and spent money they didn't have, for example, throwing a big party for Super Bowl Sunday.

"Then it was my fault for mismanaging the money when funds didn't stretch to meet. I had a lot of money sense before I met him. I knew how to save and budget. Now I was at a loss."

Another sign of abuse is watchfulness and lack of trust, and Debra had to deal with that as well.

"He was the kind of man who called all day long to check up on me. What are you doing? Why aren't you doing what I told you to do?"

She never took time for herself.

"I thought that in order to make things work, and to take care of my children, I had to devote myself to the cause 24/7. I never did anything for myself. I didn't have any friends, I had no plans, I never got my hair cut—any of those things that you can think of doing for yourself. I loved to read, but if I read, it made him mad; he said I was ignoring him. I couldn't do anything for myself without some consequence, so I devoted myself to the kids and tried to make it through this thing called life.

"My job was to keep him happy, make him satisfied, make him feel good about himself."

THE DOMESTIC VIOLENCE SPIRAL

Debra did not have the words to name what she was going through. Now she teaches others about the cycle, the predictable pattern, what is known as the three stages of the domestic violence spiral: tension, crisis, calm.

"Calm is when things seem normal, or even romantic. Tension is the build-up. Crisis is the abuse. Then it starts all over again."

There were times when he could be a good person. He could be loving, supportive, and sweet.

"He got the children special things for their birthdays without a directional prodding from me. He told them he loved them.

"He was not a terrible person 7 days a week 24 hours a day 365 days a year.

"That's what keeps bringing you back, even though in an abusive situation, when you go back, it is probably going to be worse than it was before. Every time I left and returned, it was all right for a while, which is what we term 'The Honeymoon' period. Eventually that good behavior erodes until it becomes worse than when it started."

The children could tell when it was building up. They ran out of the house and hid.

"They knew, we all knew, if he was going to explode. Get out of here! I told them. Head for the hills, that's what I called it. You knew if you were there, and he was mad, you were gonna get the brunt of it."

When you are in the middle of a situation of domestic violence, you are so busy trying to cope, you don't stop to consider, This is not right.

"You would never use the terms that we use right now about the stages, or words such as isolation, manipulation, the honeymoon, or the tension. You spend the time thinking, Well if I did this better, maybe it would stop. You lose the ability to articulate how you are feeling. You don't even think in terms of verbal or emotional abuse, it happens so gradually."

ESCALATION OF PHYSICAL ASSAULT

This is a fact: Left unchecked and unchallenged, domestic violence escalates.

"The physical assault was increasing: slapping, pushing, shoving. And one of the ways that he would abuse us was by driving recklessly: high-speed dazzling chases when he was mad."

Once, while driving, he slapped Debra so hard her glasses flew out the car window. The children were hysterical. They knew she couldn't see without her glasses. She had to walk back and get them.

X said he had a second job, but Debra never saw the paychecks, and when they called him at work he wasn't there.

"So he lied to me about that. And he was starting to be gone every Friday and Saturday night, claiming it was work, but I knew he wasn't working."

The truth is it was peaceful at home without him.

"None of us cared that he wasn't there because we didn't have to deal with his abusive nonsense. Except that we wondered what the hell is he doing? and it only takes you about two seconds to figure out he was seeing somebody else."

When one of the children was in a serious accident, and they couldn't reach him, it was the final straw. Debra told him to get out.

"He told me he was going to go stay with his mom, but he moved into his girlfriend's house. We had been married sixteen years. The children were shocked, traumatized, sad; we all were. I did not have a job, he took the only car we had. I didn't care. I'll figure it out. Enough. Enough."

POURING OUT HER HEART IN WRITING

That is when she started writing.

"Nobody told me to do it. I had never written up till that point. I just did it. My life was in crisis."

She poured out her heart, relived her frustration.

> I tried to fix things.
> I tried talking—arguing screaming crying. None of it made any difference to you.

> You continued to do exactly as you pleased.
> Finally I was worn out until I felt totally
> dead inside.

Through her writing, Debra began to realize how she closed
her eyes to the abuse when she was in the thick of it, wishing
not to see what was right in front of her. At one point, her face
had become a metaphor for unexpressed emotions.

> My body manifested my pain. Remember
> when my skin erupted in a miserable rash
> and my eyes were swollen shut? Strange how
> emotional suffering can become so physical.
> And no one knew what was wrong—what
> was the cause—because I told no one how
> inadequate I felt—how low I felt as a human
> being—not worthy of being treated with re-
> spect or honesty or love.

After he left, Debra got severe migraine headaches. That did
not make sense to her; why were they starting now? It turned
out that that is not an unusual symptom for those who have
gotten out of a dangerous situation, but have not dealt with the
aftermath.

"I had medical coverage now—I went to the doctor. She
said, You are depressed, and you have a right to be. You have a
lot to be depressed about, because of your history."

That was important to Debra, a turning point.

"She was the first doctor who actually asked the question,
Are you in, or were you in, an abusive relationship? I had been
to doctors before, and nobody had ever mentioned that. Even
when I was in the middle of a really bad abusive time, and my

five-year old was acting up, the doctor never asked. This doctor did, and she was willing to talk about it."

The doctor encouraged Debra to exercise and walk. Soon she had the migraines under control, but she was having trouble sleeping.

"Then I read *The Artist's Way* by Julia Cameron, and started writing for real."

That is where Debra got the idea for "stream of consciousness" writing. Cameron calls them "morning pages."

"I thought, 'That sounds easy, more easy than anything anybody else said to do. Empty my mind, I can do that, and it might help me sleep.'"

When Debra made writing a regular practice, something profound happened.

"Answers started appearing to things that I didn't think I had answers for."

Here again is an example of that "knowing without knowing" described in Chapter 5.

"A lot of us say, 'I don't know,' but you *do* know; it's there. I would write about things said and done, whatever was on my mind, and things would pop up. Oh that's why, and this is why."

Whenever she felt sad, Debra turned to her writing.

> Watching weddings on TLC is fun but it makes me cry. I feel like I cry all the time, and that makes me mad at me. Why do I always break down and cry? At everything and at nothing, for reasons and no reasons. Do I really want to cry? Am I angry? What is the deal?
>
> Sometimes I envy my friends who are couples. They are so happy and seem to

know where they are going in life. I don't
have that sense of self. I know more about
what I don't want than what I do want.

Some of the entries made her realize what she had been
through; things she had forgotten came back to her. And, in the
safety of her notebook, she could say to him what she could not
say face-to-face.

"Julia Cameron says have a date with yourself, so I took
myself out to lunch. At the time, I wasn't rich, and eating out
was a big luxury. I went by myself."

An ordinary moment, which, as she writes, suddenly switches.

Just had pizza buffet at Pizza Hut. I had
been wanting pizza for days! Wanting,
thinking, plotting, planning, visioning and
finally, I got it! This is a real treat. Had
salad, pizza and iced tea. Perfect lunch!

"Because my husband was a pizza delivery man, we would
get the ones that weren't delivered, or left over at night. We
were eating pizza a lot. So pizza has a role in my life."

Is it a crime to love pizza, to dream about
it? The special taste of all the ingredients
cooked together—hot crunchy moist gooey
and spicy all at the same time. Yes I love
pizza. Remember I used to crave pizza
when I was pregnant with Liz? You worked
at Smokey's delivering and sometimes you
brought home mistakes or sometimes you
bought pizza with your tips and when we

were really strapped for cash we would call
in an order to a phony address. We both
loved pepperoni pizza with mushrooms
and olives, that was the favorite. It is no
wonder Liz came out dark and spicy, the
true epitome of the Italian beauty.

Writing gets to the core. Debra starts crying.

It's making me cry to think these thoughts—
why? Maybe because those years were some
of our best times.

Now the ink and the tears are flowing fast together.

Yes they were before you got bored with
being broke and being Daddy. You started
hanging out with a friend from high school.
He was single, still had extra money for fun
things that we couldn't afford. He could
stay out all night and get as drunk or as high
as he wanted to without causing anyone
else sorrow or pain. That was not the case
for you. You had a wife, two daughters, and
two sons when you did those things, and it
did cause sorrow and pain and anger and
resentment.

It felt good to get it out. Writing was like a friend, a friend
who would listen. Whenever Debra didn't write, she later re-
gretted it.

. . . could not get to sleep last night; everything was zipping through my brain with no stopping. That means I have not been doing my writing. Don't know why I stop doing it. Things always get muddled or should I say F up when I stop writing. I need this exercise to keep my mind clear and free.

THE PERFECT JOB

Many times in her journal Debra wrote about the kind of job she envisioned for herself.

> a good job with benefits; rent paid, food on the table, and medical—when I get to that status on my own, I stop being in crisis.

She volunteered at the YMCA Shelter, and dreamt of a full-time position there.

> Working at eliminating violence grabs my attention and my heart. I simply must find a way to support myself while doing this work. It is my passion. The kind of work that gets me going, keeps me engaged and interested, satisfies my desire to help others and make a difference in this lifetime of mine. I am learning so much. About the world and myself!

Writing it down helped make it happen, and that is exactly the work she so proudly does today.

> I absolutely love my job. Working 35 hours a week at YWCA Safe Choice Domestic Violence Program as coordinator of advocacy and community out-reach. My job is perfect. I get to do lots of different things, work with women clients, supervise and train volunteers and staff, DV presentations, work with the displaced homemaker program. And I have a great boss. More than I ever expected.

Debra invites the women who come to the Y shelter to write.

"That is one of the first things that I recommend highly. I encourage the women to journal. Based on my own experience, I know it helps formulate answers."

She gives them notebooks to get them started.

"I go grab a big pile when they are on sale. 70 sheets, wide-ruled. 50 cents apiece. I bring in a stack and say, Here, take this, and use it. I know it's not pretty; you can decorate it if you want. Sometimes I bring colored paper and glue to brighten the covers."

Debra deals with women who are scared to tell their story.

"I tell them it's okay to be afraid. We are not encouraged to talk about painful things in our society."

The women think that if they don't lean into pain, they can circumvent it, and it will not hurt as much. Debra has an answer for that avoidance.

"If I meet someone who is fearful to write, I tell her I know how it feels. Do it anyway. You have to do what hurts if you ever want to get to those answers. You have to walk through the pain. You have to go through the dark scary place. Once you go through it, then you can say, I went through it. I lived through that. By writing, you can see that path clearly."

Debra tells the women that there is no one right way to write; she advises that they figure out what works for them, what helps them most, and then do that.

And she tells them they have a right to privacy.

"As a survivor of domestic violence, I know that nobody allows you to have privacy. It sounds weird to say 'allow' but if nobody encourages you to take care of yourself in any way, in fact the complete opposite, you need to spend all your time taking care of him, that's what I mean by 'allow.' There is absolutely no time in an abusive relationship that the woman would think of doing something for herself, or feel that that was allowed.

"I flat out had no privacy in the relationship. It never even occurred to me to spend time on myself. He would not have let anything be personal as far as I was concerned."

Some of the women who come to the shelter for help are still in the abusive relationship, and they are not ready to separate.

"We say, keep a journal, but be careful about privacy. Maybe you will have to keep it at your mom's house, or a friend's house, or at the shelter, a safe place. Sometimes we can't even give them our card; we can't give them our brochures. We have to say, Can you memorize our hot line number as your safety plan? When you get in a position where you need to, you can call us. Sometimes that's all we can do."

Debra tells them to write whatever is on their minds, and not to judge their words or thoughts.

"What I often find myself doing is starting out superficially."

My fingernail polish held up so well until
this morning.

Just put a load of clothes in the wash.
Changed my sheets today. Waiting for the
phone to ring.

"And if I wrote for longer periods of time, it would start to
be more real stuff, the stuff that I told myself I didn't know."

Debra is convinced that the women she works with know
intuitively what is best for them.

"They just don't think they do, because they've been told
they're stupid, that their ideas don't matter. They can't even
imagine that they can do this. They are smarter than they think."

Keep on writing, she tells them.

"Sometimes we think we don't know what we want, or
what is right for us, but if you write about it, and if you keep
working with it, you will find it."

WHY WRITE?

For Debra, there are three main reasons to write. The first is
what she calls "that déjà vu thing."

"What is it about promising yourself you will never forget
it—and then you do. Unless you write it down. If you don't
have a way to visualize it, you can pretend it didn't happen."

It might only be a single sentence of what happened, and
then you remember writing that same thing the week before.

"Then you realize, Oh my God, I've written it more than
once. Because through the act of writing it down, it sticks more in
your consciousness. The more you write, the more you notice."

The second reason to write is that journaling helps make
important choices.

Even though they were already divorced, and he was with another woman, X came over to Debra's house to tell her he still cared for her.

"It would have been so easy to give in, to have someone there to take care of things for me. I was so vulnerable, and sick and tired of doing it for myself and my four kids.

"Wouldn't it be nice to fall into somebody's arms? and live happily ever after?"

Here is where her writing helped her resolve not to let him into her life again.

"It's one thing to be convinced in a moment. If I am with him, I think he is being sincere and caring, warm and loving—which of course he would be, if he wanted to come back to me. Then after the moment goes away, it starts to feel differently.

"My journal is a place where I can talk it out. Oh, he was just here, and he said this, and this is how that makes me feel . . . This is what he said, and that's exactly what I want, too . . .

"And then I can look at it, and go over it, and reflect, You know, he said that before. And it never changes; he keeps saying it, but it never happens."

So whenever she thought she might go back to him, she used writing to resolve the ambiguity.

The best reason Debra offers for Why write? is the third one.

"Writing is something you can do for yourself. It's not expensive, and it doesn't hurt anybody, but you can gain personal benefit from it. It's cheaper than a therapist."

She laughs. "You can't afford a therapist? Write."

"For women who are abused, writing is not only therapeutic, but also pampering. You had never taken time with yourself before."

A NEW AND HAPPY LIFE

Debra does not go back and reread her journals too often, but when she does, she sees how far she has come, and how content she is now.

"I have a great life. I am happy with where I am today. I get to make all my own decisions, I have kids who are doing fine. I have grand babies, the absolute best. Great friends, great sisters, co-workers. . . ."

Life is full, from the simple pleasures. . .

> colored my hair this morning L'Oreal Color Spa #26 Redwood—it looks good!

to a whole new life plan:

> I love my classes. I have 70 credits and a GPA 3.6. I have been on the dean's list (equivalent to honor roll in high school) three times (3.75 or more), have been invited to join Phi Theta Kappa for scholastic achievement. I got a scholarship for tuition.

Last month, she took the LSATs and plans to go to law school. From an abused wife on welfare who scrubbed the mildew and stains off seedy motel shower stalls, to where she is today, Debra has come a long way.

Best of all, she is surrounded by a healthy family.

Recently, they rented a house in Sun River for the whole gang, including the grandchildren, Alex and Ashley.

It went by so fast! Bike rides, nature walks, talking, power naps. Barbecues, boating and being with each other.

Ashley has done some firsts while here with us—like laugh out loud and reach for a toy. Alex is busy trying to stand, and tooth No. 8 broke through. I got sunburned at the pool. The girls cooked breakfast. I am glad to say we did NOT turn into the Griswolds, from the Chevy Chase movie vacation.

And then, on the last night,

We ate chicken strips and fried potatoes and talked at the table until late at night.

A different scene entirely from dinner meals of the past.

What a great way to spend an evening, totally surrounded by those I love! This vacation has been so special. It feels good to be able to do this as a great big huge family group.

This is what my dream was, back when I first got together with X. That one day I would have this lovely family, this wonderful experience. And it seems that I have it! In spite of X, and without him. This is my family and I love them dearly and they love me. It is sad for me, it is making me cry, but crying is good and feeling sorry for me and

my kids is okay, too. Maybe if it happened
with him as a husband and father we could
have all been much richer emotionally and
spiritually.

"Oh well, we did achieve my dream—the long, hard, way."

Each of us is strong, loving and loved, kind,
good people. We all are moving forward in
our lives, and letting go, and growing, and
living life fully.

APPLY THIS

William Butler Yeats said, "We should write out our thoughts
in as nearly as possible the language we thought them in, as
though in a letter to an intimate friend. We should not disguise
them in any way; for our lives give them force as the lives of
people in plays give force to their words."

Use a "stream of consciousness" writing, letting your words
flow in great effusion. Start out superficially, and write unre-
strained, until you come to the knowing beneath the "don't
know."

When Debra was in crisis, she picked up her pen and did
what at the time seemed the most natural thing, and let the force
of her words run like a strong current of water along a dry bed.
You can do the same.

Pamper yourself. Write.

❧ CHAPTER 12 ❧

Branching

Getting Inside
Another's Head

Branching™ is a spiral way of organizing thoughts that I first described in *Writing on Both Sides of the Brain*. Here is how it works: Begin with the main idea in an oval or circle, and then jut out lines to indicate categories. Now add limbs to capture whatever springs to mind around the key concept. Branching organizes as it goes; it gathers like ideas together with a built-in sorting system. Where a linear, step-by-step outline cuts off the stream of new ideas as it marches relentlessly down the page, Branching keeps sections open and invites more inclusion. Branching creates a euphoria as it brings up the unexpected moments inherent in writing that flows.

In Chapter 7, you met Patti, the nurse-teacher who used writing to resolve a problem with an irresponsible student. Patti shared another writing story with me—and this time it was closer to home. When Patti had a falling-out with her younger daughter, Bianca, she used Branching as a way to find the path back to relationship, to heal the hurt between them.

Patti learned about Branching when she took a course from me years ago, and she has been using it ever since. She likes it because it parallels the way she thinks. She laughs as she describes herself.

"I am passionate, witty, creative, multi-faceted, and—I admit it—'boundary-challenged.' Branching is physically relaxing for those of us who are easily distracted. It feels natural to me, like someone has let fresh air into my room."

Patti sees Branching as a way of directing energy; she grins when she makes the connection with the non-sequential way she approaches housecleaning.

"I have a master list for all tasks, room by room, which I cut up in strips and put in a bag. Then I add a few extras, 'Read for 15 minutes' or 'Take a nap'; 'Have a coffee break'; 'Jog around the block'; 'Do sit-ups'—anything that is fun. I shake the bag up, grab one chore to do, and put the timer on for each job. I like the variety, the whimsy of it, and the fun component—why does everything have to be boring and straight-lane?

"For resolving issues, I can do linear outlines, but branching for me works better because it's more random. Branching is full of surprises. Linear outlines don't have the same energy."

THANKSGIVING WITHOUT HER GIRLS

Patti's daughters, Anya and Bianca, are in their 20s, and live away from home. Bianca is an actress making movies in Los

Angeles; Anya, a pre-vet student, is three hours north of her sister in San Luis Obispo. Patti's mother died at the end of October, and since both girls had just come home to Seattle for the memorial, they decided not to return for Thanksgiving.

"Bianca was having her sister and some friends over, cooking Thanksgiving there. At least I knew they would be with each other, but it felt odd. It was the first year we were not all together.

"My husband, my son and I took a ferry in the morning to be with my siblings on the peninsula. I made a quick call to California on my cell phone, and then the battery went dead.

"I thought they might call back later, but they didn't call all day."

That evening, there was a long wait for the return ferry, and Patti was thinking about the girls and how much she missed them.

"And I longed for my mother. I would have given my left arm to talk to her."

It was late, but Patti knew her girls would still be up, so she dialed the number. Bianca answered.

"I was so happy, she was right there. But immediately I heard in her voice that she was not pleased that I called. With a tone of annoyance she told me, 'Mom, we recorded *Friends* and we just sat down to watch it.'

"In that instant, my heart squeezed. It was a visceral hurt."

Patti said it felt like someone had punched her.

"The message was clear: the television program is more important than you are."

With wounded pride, Patti told Bianca, "Give the phone to Anya. I know she will want to talk to me."

It could have ended there, but Patti was hurt, and could not stop thinking about Bianca's snub.

MENTAL REHASH
MAGNIFIES FEELINGS

When we hold onto an imagined wrong, it festers and grows. We play and replay the scene as it builds up in intensity. We polish it, like Snow White's wicked stepmother shining up the apple. Soon, the emotions have a life of their own, a depth and severity beyond the original incident.

"When I am angry, I act. I look at options. I want to resolve it.

"When I am hurt, I withdraw."

Patti waited all day Friday for Bianca to call. She thought she was being magnanimous, allowing her daughter time to hear the tape inside her head of their brief conversation, and realize what she had done.

"I was giving her a chance to apologize. That was my way of handling it."

Bianca didn't call.

The feelings magnified. The more Patti went over the scene mentally, the more awful it felt.

"It started in my head; I leaned into feeling bad. I'm thinking, My mother has died, doesn't she realize that I am grieving? What has she learned from 9/11? She and I had had a million conversations about that, and here she is letting there be this bad feeling between us."

CONFLICT CAN BE ENERGIZING

When you are "out of relationship" and want to be back "in relationship," how do you get from here to there? Patti knew that crossing that moat of separation is hard work, and a risk. You might get bitten by an angry alligator, or drown in a swamp of accusations. You might not like hearing what the other person has to say. There is a chance that there will be things in the exchange that will offend you and cut deep. Patti understood this.

"I have taken classes in conflict resolution, and I know that no matter what the basis of the conflict is, conflict can be good, even energizing and growth-producing. People who are emotionally lazy avoid conflict because it's hard. You have to keep at it, and not give up if it gets tough.

"Conflict is uncomfortable, but if you work through it in an appropriate and reasonable manner—and there are rules for that—you can come out of it having improved, and grown, and learned through the process. But you need to approach conflict in a dedicated way depending on your relationship with the person you are in conflict with."

Patti wanted to bridge the gap between herself and her daughter quickly.

"If we let it go on too long, after a while, I won't call her to protect myself, because I am fearful that I am going to interrupt something, and maybe after a while, she won't call me because she'll think I'm thin-skinned. Or worse, she'll pick up the phone, and when she finds out it's me think, 'Oh God, here we go.' I don't want a martyr relationship with my daughter."

BRANCH #1: PATTI'S OWN FEELINGS

Patti turned to Branching as a way to sort through her swirling emotions.

"My purpose in Branching was to first accept where I was, to understand my feelings. My feelings were there and I could ignore them, or just sit with them and feed them, not understanding them. That's what a lot of people do; it takes too much work to go further."

Branching is a way of going further.

Patti's first branch looked like this:

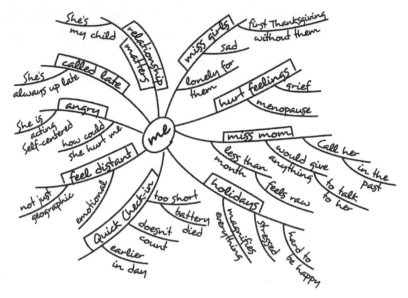

"I have gotten rid of a headache without any medication by using branching to get to the source of the pain. It gives me relief when I can see the source and say, Oh, that's what it was. I am more comfortable when I name the underlying cause.

"When Bianca didn't want to talk to me, my reaction was instantaneous, like touching a hot stove. In the moment, I was stunned, devastated. Branching helped me qualify why it stung.

"I missed my mom, I missed my daughters at Thanksgiving, and that was it: my mother, the holidays, all of those components."

Patti wrote fast without thinking or organizing by divisions. And that is an important part of Branching. You can always edit a branch or rearrange it later. Analyzing where things belong is not important, getting it out is what matters.

Patti's "Me Branch" had its desired effect.

"After doing this, I understood more of where I was, and why I felt the way I did."

BRANCH #2:
FROM BIANCA'S POINT OF VIEW

Steven Covey teaches that the most selfless act in the middle of an argument with another is to attempt the impossible: to see the disagreement through the other's eyes. Patti understood the power of this, and the toughness of it.

"I loved her enough to want to understand her side."

Patti used a second branch to explore what might have been Bianca's point of view. You cannot put yourself in someone else's head, but you can get a rough idea.

"There are things we know without knowing how we know them. I am close to her, and pick up on how she feels. The more I trust that knowing, the more frequently I get it right."

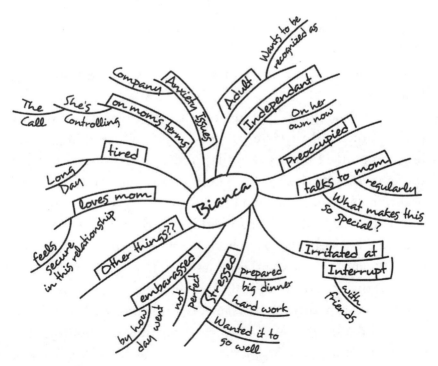

By doing this second branch, Patti had a different perspective on how Bianca might view the situation.

"Maybe she was self-conscious about how her day went. When Anya had come to the phone, she had told me that they miscalculated how long it took the turkey to cook. Kind of a hard thing to tell your mother: 'My first Thanksgiving away from you, we didn't eat until 9:00 o'clock at night because the turkey wasn't done.' If Bianca had told me that, I could have laughed with her, but maybe to her, it was a disappointment. Perhaps she had expectations for it being a home-style Thanksgiving, and it wasn't.

"When I reflected on that possibility, I was able to not have the hurt feel so physically painful."

BRANCH #3:
WHAT IS UNDER THE HURT

Before calling Bianca, Patti knew there was a third branch she had to do.

"There was something greater than just that Thanksgiving night phone call that we needed to give more thought. By branching out, I understood that under the hurt was worry. I thought, Maybe there is something else going on. The third branch helped me understand that.

"I surmised that it had something to do with her being an adult and me seeing her as a child; her wanting to be more independent, and me not wanting to let go. There were other issues too, but that was the crux of it. There had been a number of situations recently that felt the same, conversations where we felt unfamiliar at the end. We have a close relationship, but for eight or nine months, there was a distance brewing, and we had not been able to put a finger on it."

Patti did a third branch:

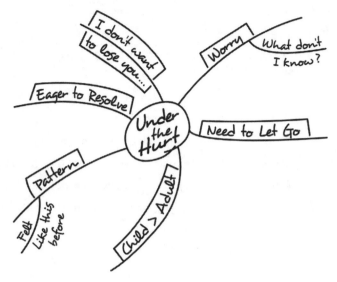

Something else came up in this last branch, a sadness and a scare Patti hadn't verbalized. She drew a line off the center and what came out was,

"I don't want to lose you."

READY FOR A PLAN

Now it was time to write a plan, a course of action, to enumerate the steps to take heal the separation between them. Patti wrote her strategy as a linear, old-fashioned list.

Plan

1. Pity Party—you deserve it (only for awhile)
2. Keep occupied and wait
3. Next time she calls, say, "Sorry, call later, I'm watching TV"

4. Talk with friends who have older children
5. Give time
6. Pray
7. Leave loving message after all of the above

She read the steps over and then wrote next to #3: "childish."

Number 4 was a concept that resonated, so Patti called some trusted friends, people who had been there.

"I didn't go to them for advice. I just said, 'My heart hurts, do you have a moment?' They didn't give me a solution. They just shared their hurts and I began to recognize how apart from her I felt."

Soon after, Patti was on the ferry again with her cell phone. She dialed Bianca.

"I intended to leave her a message, and I had rehearsed what I wanted to say: 'I've had time to lick my wounds. The world is in too vulnerable a place for us to let another day go by without speaking some loving words to each other. Even though I was hurt, I love you and I know we will eventually be able to talk to each other.' My little speech. I didn't expect her to be home."

Bianca answered the phone in person, and now they were catapulted into the confrontational conversation that Patti had been dreading. The work she had done by Branching helped her to hold her tongue and listen. Because of her writing, she had a different attitude and a different intent.

"At first Bianca was self-righteous, declaring her side. It was hard for me because I am verbal, but I shut up and let her talk. I had to actually hold my mouth closed with my hand so I wouldn't interject. It was as though she was the adult and I was the child. She was reprimanding me. My mind was thinking, How dare you? But I let her get it all out. I remembered my second branch, and instead of reacting, I responded, 'I can see how you would feel that way.'"

Bianca protested, "Mom, I already talked to you earlier that day."

Patti answered calmly, right off her branch, "It was Thanksgiving, and I missed my mom so much, and the fact that you didn't want to talk to me was more than I could bear.

"You knew I was hurt, and I banked money on the fact that you would call and apologize. As time went on, that hurt became deeper. That's what I don't understand. How could you let someone you love so much hurt for so long?"

They kept talking and soon began exploring the coolness that had been building up.

"We did a little probing. She admitted she was trying to distance herself. She said, 'Do you realize that I have been paying my own way for over a year now?' In her mind, being financially independent was the ultimate emancipation. It was a big deal for her to make enough money to do that.

"Then she told me that she wants me to trust her, to trust that whatever comes up, she can deal with it."

ESTABLISHING A CODE WORD

The willingness to continue talking next led to a valuable awareness and a change in their future interactions.

"Our line of communication had ended when I drew back after she hurt me on the phone. The conversation was over, and you can't solve anything when the conversation is over."

Bianca realized that sometimes in their interactions she was the one stewing. She called it "putting on armor" and wondered out loud if there was a code word they could come up with for one to alert the other that she was getting defensive and withdrawing.

"What she said was so true. I might say something that I haven't thought through, defending myself and she would respond in a hurtful way to protect herself. Sometimes it is the opposite, but either way, we are both doing battle and have put on suits of mail."

They decided to just say it directly, "I'm putting my armor on." Now they can recognize that whatever is going on, the other is responding in a defensive or hot way. They can step back from that, and think about it.

Patti felt a peace she hadn't felt in days. She felt closer to her daughter than ever. It was a wonderful, healing conversation. It was also fatiguing.

"When it was over, I wept for sheer exhaustion. Yet I knew that that willingness to work at it is what makes relationships that you care about solid. All this from a five-second brush-off phone call."

Well, a five-second phone call and three exploratory branches.

APPLY THIS

You may have used Branching yourself to organize your thoughts for a writing project, or gone beyond that, in a therapeutic way, to apply the random thinking to get at what is upsetting you when you can't name it. Now I am suggesting you go a step further, and see if you can use Branching to get at what is bothering another person. Be totally non-judgmental and unquestioning whether you are on target or not; write fast and without thinking or analyzing. Let the process take you where it may.

Then make a separate branch to name the worry beneath the hurt or anger, and devise a plan to resolve it.

CHAPTER 13

Vietnam Veteran

Telling His Story At Last

I've wanted to put down my thoughts about this episode of my life but was never ready. For reasons that aren't totally clear yet, I am ready now. In fact, I find the writing of this story to be necessary. I've had the images of that time in my heart for thirty-five years and now they're in my head. It's time. As I get older, I don't want to forget. I left a lot of friends behind and have a duty to remember for them. This story is not intended to make anyone feel sorry for me. It is intended to make the reader feel. If nothing else, it's a piece of what actually went on back then.

> I couldn't have imagined that I would
> be doing and having done to me the type of
> things I'm going to get into, ever.
>
> As I go through this exercise, I hope to
> uncover some of the things that still scare me.

The war in Vietnam was over three decades ago. Those who experienced it talk about it as if it just happened; it's forever fresh. Mike, an artist and a marine who served in Southeast Asia, has an explanation for that.

"You know why it's fresh? We were in Vietnam during the formative years of a person's life. I went from being a kid in Seattle to a grown man in Asia in the matter of a month. Our environment that created who we were was Vietnam, was a war. It was an ugly class. The things we did were ugly things; there was nothing pretty about it. The effect it had on us in those formative years is permanent."

Mike says there is another reason why it is fresh, and it can be summed up simply.

"There are two words that will draw a tear from any Vietnam vet. You could write a whole book around those two words. They are, 'Welcome home.'

"We were starved to hear it. But because nobody else said it to us, today we say it to each other. It is almost a code word for the brotherhood."

Recently Mike met a U.S. Senator who had served.

"I said those words to him, Welcome home. He and I looked at each other, and then fell into one another's arms, weeping. We were crying in each other's arms, understanding things that nobody else will ever understand."

Mike feels a bond with other Viet vets.

"We are family. They are my brothers. It is not quite like that with other wars. We depended on each other to survive. *When we got home.*"

ANNUAL MEETING IN ALASKA

For several years now Mike, and his buddies, Bruce, Bob, and Maynard, meet annually to talk about Vietnam, and center themselves.

"Maynard has a fourplex in Alaska. For five days, we go up there and drink too much, talk about stuff, yell a little bit, vent."

> My friends and I now get together and talk about our shared experience. We still wonder what happened. How did we make it out alive? We are not special. What we are is a group of people who survived what people call one of the worst times in our history. I'm not sure "survive" is the word I want to use. I'm not sure there is a word that covers it. Is there a word that means we went on and in most cases hid from it? Is there a word that says we forgave a lot of our country for hating us when we got back even though they haven't forgiven us? Is there a word that means we lived it but it wasn't real? If it was real, how come it's so hard to have people understand it? How come we need to stick together to talk about it? How come we can't cry?

ORGANIC AND EVOLVING WRITING

Mike is not a writer, but he felt he needed to put this down. Talking about it once a year with three close friends was no longer enough. He needed to put his memories in concrete form, in writing.

"I watched a lot of people die. I held a lot of people as they died. If I lose the memory of what went on back there, it's not fair to those people.

"Those of us who came back have a responsibility to keep those who didn't, alive."

> It seems now that all those who died couldn't have avoided it. I can't believe that Death was so accepted. That's one of the reasons why it's so important now to tell this.
>
> And those young men were fighting for what they believed at the time was a just cause.

For Mike, the writing of this memoir was organic and evolving.

"On Veterans Day one year I found the need to put some of this down on paper. I had little snippets. I decided I would do my best to document it, in one year, Veterans Day to Veterans Day. I started dumping. That's all it is. I dumped."

He put down what came to mind. The more he wrote, the more he remembered.

"I just kept writing. It didn't grow from front to back, it grew out. The original draft was eight pages. That was the base, the ground. I used that as the outline, and I would keep going back in, and adding more."

An artist, Mike has trained himself to see the entire finished picture in his head before he starts a painting.

"I can do that with the incidents in Vietnam. Although it isn't something I'm happy about. Along with the pictures in my mind come the feelings, smells and sounds."

> I sit and think and then I write. I remember the smell of diesel and gunpowder. I'm sure that most vets do. We would walk behind the trucks and tanks on maneuvers, and that smell was thick and strong. To this day, that smell can take me back to that time. The smell of gunpowder was followed by the smell of death. This type of smell usually had screams associated with it.

THE FLIGHT TO
THE SOUTH CHINA SEA

He remembers every detail of the airplane trip over, including the kindness of the stewardess, who gave him her wings as he left the plane, and wished him luck.

> It was the summer of 1968. It was a smooth flight and at the same time full of anticipation, wonder, and anger. We didn't understand the word fear yet. We were flying

Continental Airlines, heading into hell, a hell that would last inside us the rest of our lives.

We had all heard about Vietnam, most of us had lost someone or knew someone who had lost someone there. It was a mystery we needed to investigate. The plane was full of every service organization, draftees and those who had enlisted. It was a mixed bag of children becoming men with every mile, much before our time. Each of us was about to test the training we had dealing with survival. Some would survive, and a lot wouldn't.

The first stop was Okinawa. This is where Mike's first life memory took place, one he will never forget.

As we were walking toward the building I noticed a very quiet line of returning Vietnam veterans starting to board the plane I just left. It was hard not to stare at them. Their eyes were wide open. They seemed hypnotized. The movie *Platoon* has a scene just like that at the beginning.

Mike did a portrait of Oliver Stone, and spent some time with him. He thanked him for *Platoon*, especially that opening sequence. He told him he lived that. Stone said that it was one of those memories that he, and most of the veterans he's talked to, have.

Mike remembers what it was like to be among the ones arriving, and later what it was like to be one of the ones heading home.

"Every one of us who came out remembers that scene because we remember being the guys getting off the plane, and us going home. We were looking at the new guys thinking the same thing: a large portion of you aren't going to live.

"That's what the big eyes are on those of us going home. We knew they were going to die. We knew they had no concept of what they were walking into. We knew something they were about to find out, and we wished that they weren't going to have to find it out. Some of them were going to give up their lives finding it out."

SCENES FROM THE WAR

Mike was assigned to Con Thien, an outpost that sat right on the demilitarized zone, the DMZ.

> The DMZ was a strip of land between the North and South that had had all of its foliage stripped to the ground; it was also called the trace. It was flattened so we could see the enemy when they decided to come and get us. I had seen enough about that place on the TV. I began to wonder if I would ever get home. I wondered what would I be if I did get home. As it turns out we all thought the same thing.
>
> At one point during my stay there the Communists had amassed 80,000 troops, whose only objective was to destroy Con Thien and two other bases along the trace.

> We weren't told about this at the time. I'm
> happy I was ignorant of it. There was a lot
> we didn't know, for the better.

Mike shows me a video clip from a TV show done on the 25th anniversary of the war. He is crying as we watch it.

"This was filmed in Con Thien, on May 8th, 1967, the day before my 20th birthday."

Mike Wallace is telling us that forty-four died that day, all marines. At one point, he says, there were a hundred shells in ten minutes.

"The enemy kept on coming; we were a bullseye on top of a hill. Marines sitting on a forlorn hill and dying."

> With my eyes closed I can re-create that
> time. I can see myself standing quietly lis-
> tening to explosions, screams, helicopters,
> gunfire as if I were watching it on screen.
> Separating myself from reality.

His first day at Con Thien, Mike learned what the term "Incoming" meant.

> A corporal told me if I ever heard anyone
> yell "Incoming," jump in the nearest hole.
> If you were lucky enough to hear someone
> yell those words, you probably survived.
> That day he wasn't one of the lucky ones.

Once in a one-hour period they took 148 rounds of Incoming.

"This nightmare went on the entire time I was there. A lot of my friends died because of Incoming."

THE BLESSING OF DIRT AND WATER

Dirt and mud! Mike never knew until now what those words meant. He watched a tank disappear into mud during the monsoon season, into ground that was hard as a rock only a month earlier.

They lived in that mud, and came to think of it as a blessing.

> The enemy fired rockets and mortars at our position night and day. We lived in holes 6 feet down and 6 feet in (aren't you buried in a 6´ x 6´ hole?), so when a round hit close we might survive. We learned to use that wonderful mud. We spent a lot of time in it. We hid in it. A bullet can't penetrate mud as easily as it does dirt.

One day, they were getting hit, and Mike jumped into a hole half full of water and mud. Someone else was already in there.

> It was almost funny. We splashed around in there for almost an hour.

Two soldiers lived in each of these holes.

> I wonder why they never taught us about that in training? Let me tell you, living in a hole with another person, eating and reading with candlelight was a trip.

Food and water were a priority only after ammunition. There was no place to wash, and no water to wash in.

> People were dying, food was scarce and wa-
> ter (free of bugs) was not available. We put a
> tablet in our water to kill the parasite that
> was indigenous to the area. We were taught
> that the bellies on the Vietnamese women
> weren't large because they were pregnant, it
> was from a bug that was in the drinking wa-
> ter. That made you use your pills.

It was 167 days after Mike arrived in-country that he took
his first bath.

> This bath wasn't planned. It was in the Cam
> Lo River. My clothes fell off. I bent over in
> the water going from one place to another
> and that was all it took. The dirt I had been
> wearing for so long rotted my clothes off.

His first sensation was noticing how awesome the water
felt. Then he felt a little confused.

> I stood there nude, in the sun, lost. Now
> what?

The answer to that question was not what he expected.

> A corpsman came over to me. I had over a
> hundred leeches attached to my body from
> that damn river. They must've loved dirt.

"Leeches and poisonous snakes were the reason why baths
were optional."

After the leeches were all burned off me, I was able to get dressed. Showers now feel so good. I take at least one a day.

They stayed in their holes below ground at night for another reason.

A candle above ground in the night could be seen for miles. The enemy looked for that and would use those light flashes to zero in on. You would always know when someone screwed up. Incoming would arrive fast and furious at the strangest time. Sadly the person who screwed up usually didn't get a second chance to do it right.

Instinct meant learning how to stay alive.

Not lighting a match, or candle at night became instinct. I saw a lot of guys that never learned that. They died. To this day, I let instinct guide me. I meet people and right away get a feeling about that person. If it's a good feeling, I love it. If it's a bad feeling I pay attention to it.

THE FACE OF DEATH

Nineteen- and twenty-year-old boy-men could not be prepared for meeting death face-to-face.

I'll never forget the first person I held while he died. It was after one of those Incoming incidents. The first rocket in during this particular siege hit him. As I held him, another of my friends held his leg to him, it had been blown off. He was bleeding heavily and we hoped that if we held his leg on firm enough we could stop the bleeding. It didn't work. All he wanted was to get back to his family. He didn't want to leave them this way. I felt a great sense of loss because I couldn't do anything for him.

Once there was combat so close they were looking in the enemy's faces.

"A lot of people on both sides died that day. After that battle, we stopped shooting at them so they could pick up their dead."

Wagons and carts came out of everywhere. It was amazing; it was as if a battle had never happened, it was more like an accident. There was no enemy, just casualties. I wonder about that point. Was there an enemy? I know that there was a lot of killing but I didn't even know these people. That was what I understood the least. I know that after a while I was extremely angry with them all. They had killed and tortured a lot of my friends. I won't be going into the torture stories. They are too violent and if I forget those it would be all right with me. Just know that very few of us were able to escape those experiences.

PLAYING WAR ON PORK CHOP HILL

When Mike was a kid about nine years old growing up in Seattle, he and his friends played war.

> We had this hilly place just north of the Rose Garden at Woodland Park; we called it Pork Chop Hill. That place is still there. Whenever I go to the zoo, I look at that spot and remember the innocence of our war games. I believe we named it for a battle in the Korean War I had seen in a movie. A bunch of my friends and I would carry toy guns and storm that hill, we always won. We hid behind the rocks and pretended to ambush the enemy. No one ever died.

Ten short years later, it was no longer a game.

> My first ambush was nothing like the ones played at Woodland Park. I was the point man and scared to death.

He learned a lot that night about fear.

> That time in the past when we hid behind the rocks was gone. We were now hiding from actual people who wanted to kill us. Not only that, we were in the same position. We wanted to kill them. This was war.
> We took 80 percent casualties. I ran out to help; not even thinking about the bullets flying everywhere. We were grabbing guys

left and right, and running them back to the
base. I put this one guy down on the
ground; his eyes were wide open. He was
dead. That's a face I still see sometimes.

There were some pieces of his story that Mike anticipated
would be hard to read.
"I knew, because those parts were hard to write. I was beginning to uncover some of those times I'd hidden away."
Before those sections, he warns his reader.

If you're not ready, skip down a couple of
paragraphs.

He tells about days as hot as 125 degrees, and nights when the
temperature dropped to 29 degrees, and they put on every piece of
clothing they owned and slept two people to a cot for the body
heat. There is the farmer who kindly offered the parched troops
water—and put ground-up glass in it. And the girl-child with a
hand-grenade used as a human bomb. And the Tet Offensive, after
which the numbers dying went from 500 to 750 soldiers a week.
Little things influence him today. He purposely looks for
puddles to run through; he likes to listen to the rain.

I can go to sleep in a second if I hear rain. I
feel safe. I can't remember an attack in the
rain. It was as if the rain put a protective
shell around me that no one could penetrate.

He also tells some funny stories, like the one about a New
Year's Eve escapade when he schmoozed with the captain in his

tent while passing the officer's beer out, one can at a time, under the flap to guys in his squad who were poised outside.

> I knew he would never catch me, being Irish and all. We must have talked for an hour. Once I had depleted his supply of beer, I excused myself and told him to have a great New Year. As I was leaving he had something for me also; he was going to let me get away with taking all his beer only once. I've gotten better since then.

And he recalls how he started doing portraits for the soldiers, right there in the field.

> I drew pictures of their wives, girlfriends and other family members and the guys themselves. Some of those drawings were the last picture a family saw of their loved one.

INCONGRUOUS SOUNDS OF HOME

One night Mike was on watch in his hole.

> There had to be a billion stars visible. It was very quiet and I wondered what this place would be like if a war hadn't been going on. This moment was beautiful. It was the type of night that got most of us in trouble while in the back seat of the car at the drive-in.

He was listening to ham radio and picked up *The Tonight Show.*

> Listening to Johnny Carson, I jumped back home in a split second. It was so dark out that picturing a TV set screen was easy to do. For a split second I was in two worlds. I was sitting in a dirt hole, holding a loaded gun, knowing that a large number of enemies were not too far away and that they wanted to kill me. But I was also home, safe.

The next morning, as they were eating, word came down that a man in his platoon had died.

"All of a sudden, reality returned. *The Tonight Show* was for later. I never turned it on again while in-country."

Years later, Mike related that story to Johnny Carson, when he sent him his portrait.

"He seemed surprised that he was a moment of home to us. Just a moment though, that was all that was allowed."

RETURN UNDER FIRE

When Mike left Vietnam, he was 20, not even old enough to drink legally.

"I was pulled out under fire. Most people don't understand what that means, or what that was like."

Traditionally, a soldier was taken out of the field three days before his plane was scheduled to leave Da Nang for the states. That did not happen in Mike's case.

It was time to go home. We had been taking Incoming for over three days. It didn't stop long enough for anyone to move. The day my plane was supposed to leave country, I was still on the front line, and someone was still trying to kill me.

The helicopter descended, in the middle of the battle. The door gunner started grabbing the men. As my foot hit the step into the door, snipers started firing. I was thrown onto the floor of the copter. The snipers' bullets started coming in the windows of the helicopter. The windows had the glass removed beforehand just for this reason. The bullets were ricocheting through the copter. Because we were all so low, no one was hit. My face was pointing out the door, as the ground seemed to disappear. We went straight up.

He got on the plane for San Francisco out of uniform. He had the wrong chevrons on for his rank, no cover (hat), and the wrong shoes. He was still wearing the same boots he got into the helicopter with.

"I looked terrible, but didn't care. I was going home, all of us were. Just a few hours earlier, I was being shot at, and now I was on the way home."

My head was spinning. I was out and alive. What was waiting for me? I knew my childhood that I put on that plane a long time ago was not going home with me.

What and where and who was I going to be?
That is a question I'm still trying to answer.

Mike landed in Seattle around 7 A.M. No one was there to
meet him. He brought himself home from the airport.

> I caught a taxi and came home. There was
> no debriefing, no fanfare, no parades, just
> the long cab ride. The shock of that is still
> with me.

He could hardly believe he was home and safe. He needed
to see if it was real. He walked over to the university campus.

> As I reached the freeway overpass, I walked
> right into a protest against the war. That was
> the first time I was called a baby killer, the
> first time I was spit at, and the most scared I
> had been in a long time. What was happen-
> ing? Where did my home go? Why did these
> people hate me? How could I cope with all
> of this, I still had friends dying over there.

He went back to his apartment terrified.
"And then I learned to shut up."

NORMAL LIFE, WOULD IT EVER BE?

He was still a young kid, and tried to go back to ordinary life.
"I went to a party where I met a girl who said her fiancée
served at the same place I did, and would be coming home soon

for their wedding. I couldn't look at her. I didn't want her to know that I had loaded what was left of him in a helicopter and read his dog tag."

> I left the party right away; I couldn't be the
> one to tell her.

A shocking statistic surrounds the high rate of suicides among those who fought in Southeast Asia. Fifty-five thousand Americans, mostly military men, died in Vietnam. Over 150,000 vets have killed themselves since they got back. Mike says he is no psychologist, but he thinks he has an explanation for that.

"There was nowhere to go. Think about this. You're a kid, you've been scared out of your wits. You've been a part of something for a long period of time that has shocked your entire system, changed who you are. The only thing we talked about—you'll hear this from every Vietnam vet—we all knew how many days we had left, every day. Before we could come home."

His voice cracks, and he pauses, overcome with emotion.

"You get frightened to death, and all you can think about, like a little kid, is getting home where it's safe. So you get on that plane to come back. You have survived the ultimate horror. You come home, and everybody hates you. Your family has changed, your girlfriend's gone, your job's gone, you have very little education. Nobody wants to hear your story. There isn't anybody who wants to put an arm around you and say, It's okay. Even the other veterans can't talk to each other because of the same feeling.

"So for years you had to carry it yourself."

And for some, it was just too much to bear.

For Mike, writing about it has helped. Even though it brings back painful memories, it underlines the contrast with today.

"I have a pretty nice life. Wonderful friends, people who love me, and whom I love. Got a great job and a strong religious belief. God is with me all the time. I have no particular religion that I practice, it is personal thing. I'm okay. I am sitting here telling a story to you.

"There is a reality that I am aware of: I *am not there anymore.*"

ATTRIBUTES LEARNED
THAT ARE PART OF HIM TODAY

Being a marine in war gave Mike attributes that serve him well today. He wouldn't say he is fearless, but he has a great deal of confidence in what he can accomplish, and especially in what his art can accomplish.

"I've drawn pictures of sixteen hundred celebrities, including some of the toughest people you could ever imagine in your life. I have made the mistake of being shy and reserved and lost opportunities. I am not asking anybody to do anything that isn't wonderful, so I have conviction in what I'm doing. I am prepared for them to say no. I'm not going to be crushed, it's not the end of my world. But if I don't ask, I don't give them a chance to say yes."

WHY HE DRAWS

Mike came back thinking there had to be something better than war. Art allows him to go someplace better.

I wonder what I would have been like without this episode in my life? Would I care as much about people as I do? Why was I spared? I'm doing some things now that are meant to thank God for bringing me home.

"I do things that try to make people feel better. I read in the newspaper about a father whose two daughters died in a car accident. I did a portrait of the girls. It helped him to let go."

I know how important the picture of those two little girls was for the family. That knowledge came from the realization that the images drawn in Vietnam were important. I put myself in the place of the family.

Not everything I came back with was bad if that ability is the product of that time.

Mike has raised $1.5 million for charity with his artwork.

I believe I was brought home to help raise those funds. I once told a reporter that I've been given a gift, and I hope I'm doing what I'm supposed to be doing with it.

He gets sad and suddenly solemn.

"I have watched life go out of people. What kind of responsibility is that? Does the spirit disappear, or do we pass it on? I think we pass it on."

WHY WRITE?

Mike showed some early pages of his Vietnam memoir to a friend who is a professional writer. Meaning well, the fellow marked it up and suggested changes.

"We are good friends and I appreciated that he was trying to help, but I didn't want somebody to read this to correct it. I wanted somebody to read it to listen, to hear it.

"I was satisfied with what I had intended to do. I didn't care about the grammar or structure. I wasn't trying to write a short story or book. I was trying to put it down."

> I am different now than I would have been without this experience. Just writing this down is changing me. It's allowing me to see what helped build me.

It was not his plan to edit it or publish it. He wanted to put it in a form where he could share it with family and friends.

> This is a piece of me that you should know.

"I felt better after I wrote it. It felt good to get it down. Writing it allowed me to break free. And once I wrote it, it allowed others to know my experience."

RECONNECT: PLEASE TRY

Mike has a direct message for the few close friends and family members who have read his whole manuscript. He understands how difficult it must be for them to understand.

I can't imagine that we went through that. If it's hard for me and I lived it, how much harder it must be for you. It is important that you try. There's a connection that I believe was broken, and most of us only want to reconnect. We aren't looking for sympathy, what we are looking for is recognition for those of us that didn't come home and their families. So please try.

As he writes down these incidents, Mike begins to understand himself more, and it helps explain why some days he can wake up happy and then have a wave of sorrow come over him for no apparent reason.

Imagine the torment if you were sad, and couldn't figure out why. All of us who were there feel sad periodically. If we understand the reason why, we can deal with it. Thank God I have some of that ability.

Mike has one key piece of advice for anyone who wants to write.

"Just start."

Once you start, writing takes on a life of its own.

"You become connected, and then you find time. You can't plan ahead; it's an emotional thing. If it's important enough, you'll start it. Get into a discussion with yourself and put it on paper so you know what you said. Don't worry about your writing style or about your spelling. Only go as deep as you want."

Writing has allowed him to break free in a way that talking about it never did.

This is something that I feel compelled to write about. Its only intention is to keep me from forgetting. It's too important for that. It has shaped a great part of who I have become.

"Thanks to Vietnam, I understand death and dedication and I know what life is about."

APPLY THIS

Consider writing a memoir about an important event in your life. Not for publication, but for yourself, to name what shaped you, and perhaps to share with a few select close friends and family members. Mike told the people he shared his story with, "If you want to understand me, here it is—this is what I went through."

Be honest, write continuously, without worrying about style or grammar. The more you write, the more you will remember.

Just start.

CHAPTER 14

A Matter of Containment

Writing and Ritual

Connie Sue divorced her husband when his verbal abuse became physical. After she left, she had to redefine who she was.

"I was no longer a Miss, I was no longer a Mrs. I was now a survivor of domestic violence. What does that mean? And how can I continue? And offer strength to other women?"

For Connie Sue, finding the answers to these questions is where writing came in. And she combined her writing with ritual to make what she felt more concrete.

When I met Connie Sue at Barnes & Noble, the first thing I noticed about her was that she was dressed all in pink, including her sneakers. She laughed lightly and explained it was her special color and her new nickname: Pinkly.

She had a story to tell me.

One of the sad truths of domestic violence is that it can strike anywhere. Connie Sue lived in a fancy house on a golf course with a large deck for entertaining. There was a three-car garage with a heated driveway; walk-in closets and a jacuzzi in the master bedroom. It was hard for her to get people to believe what was happening behind the etched-glass double door entry.

As a young girl, Connie Sue was vivacious and smart. She had many friends and traveled a lot.

"I was independent, and financially able to take care of myself—that was important to me."

She had just turned 30 when they first started dating.

"He was charming and sophisticated, and fourteen years older. He was my boss. I thought it was a very romantic relationship. He had been married two times before, and had three children. I liked the idea of a ready-made family. I thought I had met Mr. Right."

During the ten years they were together, he continued to climb the ladder as a national sales manager. They lived a luxurious lifestyle.

"I absolutely wholeheartedly believe that this person adored me, and loved me. He did not set out to want to hurt me. He was attracted to my strength, my career, my charisma, and my ability to talk to people."

A VISUAL SIGN:
THE IMPRINT ON THE WALL

When they were dating, he blew up a few times. She blamed it on alcohol.

Then at their wedding reception, still in his tuxedo and she in her bridal dress, he exploded at her in front of all the guests.

She made excuses for him, dismissing it as being connected to drinking, and all the expectations of the perfect wedding.

But deep down, she was shaken.

"I thought, 'O my God, what did I just do?'"

Within a week after they got back from their honeymoon, he told her she was no longer to work.

Now that Connie Sue volunteers, with Debra, to help other women get out of abusive situations, she knows that financial control is one of the signposts of domestic violence. Connie and Debra use a wheel, divided into pie shapes, to alert women to the patterns. The triangle labeled Economic Abuse describes Connie Sue's life to a T: "Preventing her from getting or keeping a job, making her ask for money, giving her an allowance, not letting her know about or have access to family income."

Connie Sue also knows now that what starts out as emotional and verbal abuse becomes physical abuse; name-calling and yelling lead to shoving, pushing, choking. Then it starts building.

"The escalation of the physical abuse is what woke me out of what was happening. Now it was real. I was slammed into the dining room wall, which made an indentation in the plasterboard, the outline silhouette of my body. The imprint was something visual I could see every day and realize what was going on."

HOW IT GOT TO THAT
POINT: WORTHLESS AND ASHAMED

Connie Sue's husband had rigid role expectations, again a classic warning sign.

"My entire week revolved around making the house and the yard perfect, getting ready for the next entourage of business associates to entertain, perhaps preparing to go on a business trip with him. There was an impeccability of decor and setting in place. I was to prepare the environment, and take care of food, alcohol, barbecues. When he came home from work, the idea was to have dinner all ready and a cocktail in hand."

In return, she got tirades.

"He often shouted at me, 'This is my house. If you don't like it, get the F out. I am the king of this castle.' Over and over, banging his fist down, 'My house, my money, I work, mine, mine, mine, mine, mine . . . ' and I started believing it. I felt worthless."

They lived next to a golf course, but she was not allowed to golf.

As Debra pointed out earlier, it may be hard to understand that word, "allow" between adults.

"The repercussions were too great if I did something he didn't like. I would not risk it most of the time; it would be too heavy a price to pay."

If she exercised, he suspected she might meet some men.

"Whenever I went to the gym or did anything good for myself, he accused me of messing around, of having an affair."

In the pie chart, this is a form of isolation: limiting outside involvement, using jealousy to justify actions.

Connie Sue wanted the marriage to work, and did everything within her power to make it work. She was physically worn out by the constant worrying: "What can I do to make this better? What can I do to make this person happy?"

She left several times—the average is seven to ten times a woman will leave before she leaves for good. Each time, she had it planned out.

"When I went, I took a paper sack, a blender and a mini coffeepot. I would shower at the gym, sleep at the rest stops, and plug in the blender in an outlet and live off Slim Fast, that was my sustenance.

"I slept at the rest stop many times."

But every time, she came back, blaming herself.

"Then I said, it must be me. I will try harder, clean house better, be a better wife, make everything perfect for when he comes home. I promise I won't make Hamburger Helper again."

With perspective gained through distance, Connie Sue can explain:

"What looks to others like the inability to make a decision or pure stupidity is not; it is gaining knowledge and resources of what we need to make a final decision.

"Every time we leave and come back, we get a little bit smarter and a little bit stronger."

BACKHANDED ON HER
BIRTHDAY: THE FINAL STRAW

An incident the night of her birthday brought things to a head. She had purchased herself a year membership in the local gym. He was so infuriated by this innocent act that he took the checkbook and slapped her face hard with it. He said, "That is your f—ing birthday present, and that's all you're getting."

This time Connie Sue did something she had never done before.

She called the police.

Connie Sue recalls how Nicole Brown Simpson, in a journal released after her death, described O. J.'s facial transformation when he was angry with her.

"That is exactly what my husband looked like that night I called the police, I swear to God. He was screaming at me, he had gone into my purse, and he was standing there in a fury, so mad that the veins in his neck were protruding. It was the exact same scenario Nicole depicted: he was beet red, and his eyes were bulging."

She starts to act it out now; her voice drops menacingly. Enunciating every word, grinding her jaw, she speaks with a low, slow voice as though she is telling a heart-pounding ghost story.

"Like this, 'Don't you ev-errrr . . . don't you ever dare to do anything like that again.'"

And then he hit her.

"I turned around, picked up the phone, and said, 'I've been assaulted by my husband.'"

By the time the police got there, the picture was much different than what had just happened.

"He was gracious, courteous. Mr. Calm. Mr. Millionaire. A pillar of the community. I was the one hysterical."

The police took in his polite demeanor, the appearance of the home, and the fact that at the moment Connie Sue did not look hurt. Her lip had been cut from the inside, but the bruise and the swelling weren't visible until the next day.

"The only person who is crazy, the only thing out of place was ME."

In a placating way, the police told Connie Sue, "Your husband has agreed to leave for the evening. We're not going to arrest him. He's going to get a hotel."

The police are sometimes trained on these matters, sometimes not.

A year later, Connie Sue was given an opportunity to be part of a program of police re-education, to talk about the incident to the County Sheriff's Department.

"I went in with another volunteer who had the opposite experience, where they did make an arrest, and it made all the difference."

The police did not know it was not as easy as cooling off in a hotel for a night.

He came back to the house the following morning in a rage, furious that she had called the police.

"I knew at that moment I had to leave. He could have killed me: he was that angry and that crazed."

Remembering now, she starts to cry, and bites her bottom lip. Her voice is soft, almost a whisper.

"I swear to God, I thought I was going to die. The look on his face still haunts me."

That was the day that she left for good. She went to Safeplace, a woman's shelter.

PEOPLE ASK, WHY DID YOU STAY?

People looking in from the outside, not understanding the complex dynamic of spousal abuse and domestic violence, often ask the victims incredulously, "Why did you stay?"

There are many different answers to that unthinking question. For Connie Sue, now Pinkly, part of it was psychological. She had no self-esteem. Because she cared about him and loved him, she says, she trusted him with her weaknesses as well as her strengths; he took advantage of that, and rather than building up her strong points, he emphasized her failings.

"When I was with him, I didn't like myself at all. I absolutely one hundred percent was brainwashed to believe that I could not live without this person. He took away my confidence, my vivaciousness. He was like a vacuum, 'I am going to suck you dry.'"

She freely admits that another factor was financial.

"There's no shame for thinking, 'Wait a minute, this is a good lifestyle. If I leave, I'm going to be giving this up. What am I going to do?'

"Up to the point that I had married this person, I had done extremely well for myself. Now I wasn't working. I had adjusted and become accustomed to this way of life. I was a caretaker at home, keeper of the family ties, including his children—I got along well with them. If a woman decides she doesn't want this anymore, she has to give all that up."

> If I leave, what will I do, where will I go,
> how will I take care of myself? I have no
> money, I have no job, I have nothing. Who
> would believe me?

And she also thought, "This is my home too. I have put my creativity, my personality into this home."

> Leaving behind me what I truly love, caring
> and tending to the garden. The enormous
> amount of joy it brings to myself and others.
> The golfers yelling over the fence, "Look at
> all her flowers, how beautiful they are."

And then there were parts that were good about him. As Debra says, no one is mean 24/7.

"That's what you keep hanging on to, you keep believing that the goodness will compensate for the cruelty."

But ultimately, Pinkly has an answer for those who ask judgmentally, Why didn't you leave?

She tosses her head back defiantly: "I *did* leave."

When she got to Safeplace, she bought herself a journal, and began by writing that sentence over and over. Then she went back and put it in big letters in triumphal exclamation adorning the inside cover:

"*I did leave!*"

A CONTAINMENT
FOR LEGAL DOCUMENTS
AND COURT PROCEEDINGS

Leaving, it turned out, was only the first step.

"Because of the control he had over the finances, the home, and its contents, I was re-abused through the legal system for the next four years."

Wanting this over.

Deposition tomorrow

Be strong, brave, articulate. Think before talking, answer slowly, pause, consult with attorney if need be. Feel positive, truth will prevail.

Honest, truthful, strong. Do not be defensive!

A solid week since the deposition pure depression

Walking in a daze

Another legal chapter.

Please God let it be the end.

When it was finally over, she wondered what to do with all the paperwork accumulated, the motions to compel, the discovery requests, the legal documents of literally dozens of court appearances, some of which might be important later on.

"I find containment extremely helpful. I needed a place to put it."

> Monday I finally got my last legal docu-
> ment from the uncoupling of XYZ. Bought
> a plastic box from the hardware store and
> had a little ceremony.

"I filled this huge, thick, white storage box with nothing but legal papers. I set it on the table and put a bouquet of flowers on top of it, with two candles at either end. I had a burial about legal proceedings.

"My little symbolic rite was not to dispose of it, but to contain it, get it into a single area, and put it away."

She took a picture of the filled box and the candles and pasted the photo in her journal, and then wrote about it.

STARTING NEW: AND PINK

The day Pinkly moved out of the shelter into her little one-bedroom apartment, she penned an outpouring of emotions with no logic or connection.

"It didn't matter. It was good therapy to just dump it all out."

> Uncoupling from an abuser
>   Anger feeling betrayed
>   Validation
>   Not believe, made up (like you thought
> I made this up?)
>   Depression sets in—everything seems
> overwhelming
>   Fear of the unknown
>   Back to the basics . . .
>   This is not your fault

You do not deserve this!

The jumble of words in fact was teaching her something not only about writing but about herself.

"I always thought journaling had to be perfect. It had to make sense, you had to have all your commas and periods and so on and so forth—but it doesn't."

Pinkly was used to writing on a computer with spell-check and grammar programs. At first she was worried if she wrote on a piece of paper, she would not catch the mistakes.

"Oh my, what if somebody reads what I write and it's not perfect?"

Inexpensive drugstore notebooks freed her in more ways than one.

"Spiral notebooks didn't have to be perfect. What did that say about me? I didn't have to be perfect either."

Eventually, she got brave enough to try different sizes and shapes and fancy fabric-covered books.

Pinkly now does what before would have been unthinkable. She leaves blank pages, and, if the mood strikes her, starts a new journal altogether.

"I like different journals for different thoughts. I don't have to fill a whole journal. I can leave pages blank, let them be empty, and go on to something else. I had to convince myself that that was okay; after all, leaving empty space is not perfect!"

In addition to her writing, she often includes photos and memorabilia, scrapbook style.

"My first decoration that I hung up was a paper towel and this is it. It is captioned *Things that make you happy*—and printed with cartoon pictures of puffy clouds, cuddly dogs, flying a kite, ice cream, hot cocoa, good friends, etc."

This ordinary kitchen convenience had added meaning. To her it was a sign of hope. A new beginning. Next to the illustrated sheet, she writes:

> In the grocery store, I stumbled across the same paper toweling they had at the shelter.
>
> Where it started, it begins anew. From the moment I found this, I knew there would be life again. All things are in my reach again—work, school, friends, family, and endless opportunities—what I have desired and more than I could ever dream of.
>
> From a single sheet of a papertowel found at Safeplace, I now make my own sanctuary of peace, my own safe place!
>
> I am safe at last.

MAKING 800 SQUARE FEET FEEL LIKE HOME

With her husband, Pinkly had lived in a beautifully designed and elegantly landscaped executive home, 2,500 square feet, with a cook's kitchen, and two fireplaces. The realtors billed it as "resort living every day of the year." Pinkly had a different description:

> It was a grand house but an empty house.

Her new place is only 800 square feet, but it feels both serene and strong. Part of the reason for that is her unusual decorating scheme.

"I did it positively in the 'power of pink.' I have matching pieces, curtains, and other accessories in pink."

Keeping everything within one color range gives the small space a larger feel.

But where did the pink come from? In her journal, the answer is first an exultation.

Out of nothing, comes pink!

More thoughtfully, she explains, "When one leaves with nothing in the hand, you take with you only what is in your heart. Pink came out of my spirit that this person wasn't going to break me; it was the only thing I could grasp onto. It wasn't monetary, it wasn't something that I could hold; it was something I could feel. I didn't plan for it to happen, it just kind of evolved. Concentrating on a single color makes a soul statement without being angry. People who come in contact with me, remember that. They know that I am a survivor. I talk about it, and I don't have to be angry.

"Pink has made my life simple. Everything goes together, and I am not confused by a lot of colors and choices. It's pink, or variation of pink."

A RESTING PLACE

As Jan describes in Chapter 2, death and divorce are parallel, the emotions the same. That is true especially when you are coming out of an abusive marriage. One of the more resourceful and dramatic actions Pinkly took was finding a physical place for her sorrow.

"I was in agony because I was experiencing a death, and I didn't know how to articulate that, or how to share it."

> Where do I go from here and dear God,
> what do I do with all this pain? God, I need
> help. I need direction. The pain is unbear-
> able; so deep, there are no more tears left to
> cry. It must be released, and then I must
> find a place to put it.

"It was to the point where I felt I was dying myself. It was excruciating. Finally, I went to a cemetery and walked around. I searched until I found a grave marker with the same name as my married name."

The information about the individuals interred was on one side of the tombstone, and the family name on the other side.

"That was fine, that was all I wanted—my former last name on a large granite slab. I would visit that a lot. And do my writing."

> Can I leave all fear where one goes to grieve?
> Yes, this is a place, it is right. A place where
> my thoughts are not distracted, where I can
> focus on God, write, and go on. . . .

She put meaningful objects on the surrounding ground, and took pictures to paste in her journal. First, balloons.

> Balloons at the graveside, one for each year
> I was entrapped.

"The potted geranium: I was an avid gardener. The flowers are dead. I was going to throw this plant away when I was in the process of moving, but it held a symbolic connection. The high-heeled shoe and the tiara crown represent the Cinderella Complex that I grew up with, not having a father. I never knew my father."

Her last trip to the cemetery was after her divorce papers were final.

> I've come back to where I came almost two years ago, but there are no tears, only deep deep sighs of relief.
>
> Just taking the time to write again feels wonderful. The cemetery with the head-stone, a springtime rain cleansing the soul.

"What is awesome about it is that if I get sad, I can go back there. I can mourn over this marriage in a tangible way."

LEAVING IS NOT
A ONE-TIME EVENT

Leaving an abusive relationship is a process, not a one-time event. Pinkly is adamant about that. You have to keep mentally leaving, she says, and then leave again, and leave again, and leave again. It's not something you do once, it is not a single episode but a series.

"There is not a band-aid that fits over the wounds when you put a woman in a shelter. There is so much rethinking and rebuilding of your personal self-esteem."

> Will I ever heal from feeling worthless?

"Talk about Ground Zero, no kidding."

Pinkly notes how the national tragedy of 9/11 raised our awareness about post-traumatic stress disorder, or PTSD. The symptoms are real after total destruction, even if you survived. And you need to take care of those symptoms.

It's like standing by helpless as your home burns to the ground.

"Imagine there was absolutely nothing you could do about it; you were not allowed to go back in, and there was not a firefighter around to put out the flames. What kind of sensations and emotions would you go through? You just watched as literally your whole life was destroyed in front of you.

"How would you possibly rebuild your life?"

That's how lost and devastated she felt.

This perspective makes her sympathetic to women who return.

"I tell you I would never ever ever judge a woman if she went back to her abuser. Would not. Ever. Because I understand the reasons why she would go back. It's not easy to give up your whole existence. I left. Now what?"

It wasn't supposed to be this way; wait a minute—you didn't tell me it was going to be like this.

"Just being able to state that eased my mind."

In her journaling, she wrote true things to herself.

"That was important. To be honest with myself, even if it hurt. The tears that I cried as I wrote were painful, but I understood that in order to go through to the other side, I had to get past that pain."

She stumbles over her words, trying to explain the inexplicable.

"I was brought up to believe that everything had to be neat and tidy; we are not supposed to hurt."

Writing is an end in itself. It doesn't take away the ache, it simply acknowledges it.

"When you write, there doesn't have to be any kind of result. The pain doesn't have to go away; it may not even get better. You may cross to the other side, or you may not, or it may take awhile. Writing is a way to just *be* with it, be with your pain, or your sorrow, or whatever it is. It is okay to hurt, to feel sad. And maybe you can expound on that in your journal."

For Pinkly, even carrying a journal brings serenity. It's like a kind companion walking with you in silence.

"I get comfort just from holding it. I don't necessarily have to write in it."

She carries a small portable chair in the trunk of her car.

"Sometimes I pull over, and put out my little fold-up lounge chair. I look for green space, a park, or maybe the beach; water is good. And I write."

HELPING OTHER BATTERED WOMEN

When Pinkly was living in that grand but empty house, she felt alone. Now she is part of a group that cares, and understands.

"I thought this had never happened to anyone before. And then when I found out differently I thought, Well how come I didn't know?"

So she set out to teach others.

"I learned how to be supportive of women in abusive relationships. Number one, is: Believe them—don't minimize, don't deny, don't judge. Just listen and support.

"You don't have to fix it. Just be supportive."

Validation is key.

"Give them some worth and consideration, because they haven't had that for some time."

It is an educational process, informing and letting women know how verbal abuse and emotional abuse escalate to physical abuse.

"And to let them know there are things that you can do. And you can feel crazy without being crazy."

Today I gave myself a gift.
I loved myself again.

WHY WRITE?

Writing has helped heal Pinkly. And there is another reason why she believes it is important for her to document what took place with her.

"It's history and it needs to be told. This is what happened. Even now in my life although the environment is safe, I still face pain, and financial struggles. When you have this kind of background, when you've worked through this kind of trauma, it's okay to feel sad. When I read what I wrote, I have to sit back and say, God, it's okay to feel sad today . . . it's okay to feel mad . . . it's okay, you know?"

She bites her bottom lip, starts to cry, and continues the litany, as though reassuring herself.

"It's okay if I get depressed. It's okay.

"And then I'll write some more."

Pinkly likes journals with quotes included, "because other people have written in them already.

"And maybe all I need from this particular journal are what others have said, or the artwork."

She selects a journal that looks half-empty.

"You might think I didn't use it. I have picked this book up umpteen times just to look at quotes."

The important thing, she says, is that a journal, any journal, is a container. It contains her voice.

"Even if no one else hears it, at least I hear it. I guess that's why I do it. When I write, I remember my story, and that raises the bar for other people to do what I did safely, whereas before they may not have had that choice.

"It wasn't in my personality before; I didn't have a voice, and now I have a voice."

> It is a new season. Plant new seeds carefully, tend to the new growth, use caution when weeding so as not to discard what may be sprouts of new life.

APPLY THIS

Find a color that is your spirit. Find what moves you when you write. Paste in photos and quotes from others. Be creative in journal writing, whatever that creative process is. It doesn't have to be perfect.

❧ CHAPTER 15 ❧

A Serious Disease

Living Each Day Fully

Zig Ziglar and other motivational gurus speak about the importance of an "attitude of gratitude." For my friend Jane, paying attention to the positive was more than a platitude. She says it helped save her life.

Jane and I sing in a choir together. Even though she is a soprano and I am an alto, we often wind up singing next to each other, right in the middle where the two sections meet. She heard I was writing book about healing, and one night after rehearsal, we stood in the dark parking lot for a long time, talking. Until that night, I didn't know that Jane had been in the Peace Corps in Africa, had lived in France, and has a son who was born deaf. Until that night, I did not know that Jane was a survivor of lupus. Writing, she told me, was part of the package that helped her get well.

We could have talked for hours, but it was getting cold, so Jane invited me to come for lunch at her house the following day to continue our conversation.

JANE AND IIER SONS

When I arrived, Jane put on a pot of fresh coffee, and set out on the table slices of pumpkin bread a neighbor made. We sat on the sofa looking out into her yard, watching the robins play at the birdbath and tug at worms, as she told me more of her life story.

With a mother's intuition, she sensed from the start that something was wrong with her firstborn son, Frank.

"The hardest part was waiting for the professionals to confirm what I already knew; they dismissed me as an overanxious parent or told me he was retarded."

When Frank was 15 months old, she finally found an audiologist who diagnosed his severe hearing loss, and started his rehabilitation.

Then her second boy, Tom, was born with cleft lip and palate.

"The baby couldn't come home with me from the hospital; he had to have the first of many, many operations. I felt very sad. From that point on, it seemed as though my life consisted of two things: deaf clinics and surgery."

TIRED ALL THE TIME

Tom was a good runner from the time he was young. He and his mom entered 10K races together. Jane enjoyed these meets.

"I even won a turkey once, in a Thanksgiving race. Up until then, I ran just for fun; that time, I glanced around and realized that in my category, between age 30 and 40 years old, I was ahead of everybody. I thought, 'I could even win this.' And then I ran to win, and it was neat because I don't remember ever going for the gold like that."

Jane got better and better at running, finally completing a marathon.

"Then one day, I went on a race, and I couldn't even finish it, I had to quit. I knew something was wrong."

She thought she needed to rest, to get away.

She and the boys went on a trip to Southern California to visit friends in San Diego.

"We would do something like go to the zoo, but I was just so tired, I would lie down in the sun and collapse, and let them run around and see the animals. Then we would go to Marineland or Sea World, and the same thing would happen. I rested, and let them go do the sightseeing. A few days of that and I was very, very sick."

She thought it was probably the flu, but when she got home, she broke out in a rash that looked like animal bites on her arms.

"I didn't know what that meant, but I happened to run into my ex-husband at the bank. I told him I had been feeling rotten, and that I had dermatitis. He was a doctor himself, and he suspected immediately what was wrong. He looked at me and said, 'You'd better go see your doctor.'"

She did, and that's when she was diagnosed with lupus.

THE DISEASE

Jane explains as simply as possible.

"Lupus is autoimmune disease, the opposite of AIDS or cancer. Instead of having no immunity, your immune system produces too many antibodies."

Normally when there is an inflammation, antibodies try to kill the infection, the virus, the bacteria. They know what they are supposed to kill.

"In an autoimmune disease, the antibodies get their signals mixed up and somehow attack good healthy cells. It can be show up in different places; lupus is not confined to the joints, like arthritis, but can be anywhere."

Medical students are told, "Know lupus and you know medicine." That is because it affects every part of the body, and gives a clue to understanding how the human immune system functions.

Jane told me that the word "lupus" means "wolf," and thus the bitelike marks on her arms were an indicator. She explained that the disease can vary a lot from person to person.

"With some people, it affects their skin; other people, their joints or heart. The main thing about lupus is that it always makes people who have it fatigued."

The serious part for Jane was that the lupus was attacking her kidneys, and she thought that they were going to fail.

"The doctors told me that half the people with my condition would be dead within five years."

MAGIC MOMENTS

Jane felt totally overwhelmed, caring for her boys with all their problems, and now battling a life-threatening disease herself. And then she started to write.

"I don't know how it began, but every morning, I got out my old manual Smith-Corona and typed out ten what I called 'Magic Moments,' in order to look on the bright side. It got to be a ritual, something I did every day."

- Working together with Dottie on weeding
- Dogwood magnificent
- not needing aluminum hydroxide
- the birds that keep on singing

"I made myself do ten, even if I didn't feel like it. I always felt better after. It was like meditation or exercise."

- party at Trudy's
- opportunity to get something nice, a gift for my friend
- the lush green fields
- my mind that wants to know how tulip fields are managed
- Saturday coming
- Terri willing to come look at the front yard

"After I was released from the hospital, there was a time I was staying with some friends on Lake Sammamish. I could hardly do anything, but I dragged myself down to the lake, and made myself swim every day. It felt like healing waters, it was so good for me."

Writing the Magic Moments was like that.

"It could be little things, like realizing that my yard was full of worms and the birds were there getting fed in my garden, and the tulips were coming up. Also cute little sayings my kids would come home with."

The disease dragged on, and Jane's kidneys were not getting any better; in fact, they were getting worse. The doctor told her that she might have to go on kidney dialysis, or else have a transplant. That scared her into getting chemotherapy.

"My hair was falling out from chemotherapy, my face was swollen from cortisone drugs and steroids; I was a wreck. What saved me was friends who saw me as beautiful. And I wrote."

She kept it up like medicine, ten a day.

"Whatever helps emotionally, helps physically. I definitely believe that, especially with a stress-related disease."

A SWITCH IN THINKING

The ten magic moments did something to cause a shift: a shift in attitude, a shift in outlook, and it would carry through for hours.

Jane started to focus on what was right, to appreciate her boys more, and to stop worrying about them.

"I let Frank be more independent, let him go on his own more, which he needed, instead of looking after him so cautiously. It's not good for kids if their parents are anxious about them."

Before, she was afraid that others would tease Tom because his nose and mouth weren't perfect.

"One day, while in the city on errands, I noticed a young man walking toward me at a distance. What a nice-looking guy—tall, dressed just right, I thought. As he came closer, I realized it was Tom! What a handsome fellow."

That day, she saw him through different eyes than she had been seeing him.

"I had been focusing on what was wrong, not the whole person.

"That was a magic moment."

- Tom looked so handsome to me today when I saw him on the street, and he didn't know I was looking at him.

Jane started paying attention to what her sons were doing right, and she felt proud of them.

- Tom repaired his car.
- Frank looking sharp in his new shirt.

- Tom calls thoughtfully to tell me Steve is "kind of alone" and wants him to stay for dinner.
- Frank and his friends are good company.

LEARNING FROM HER SONS

Jane admired her sons' approach to their own medical problems and learned a lesson from their upbeat attitude. Tom had many operations, including, as a teenager, major surgery where they took a bone out of his hip and rebuilt his jaw. To compound it, he had serious diabetes when he was 16.

"He was in the hospital and I worried so much about him. He did recover, and continued with sports. In the fall, he was in a cross-country race. I was concerned because he wasn't in the front of the pack—he wasn't one of the winners.

"But what did he do? After the race, he came to me and said, 'Mom! did you see my lead?!!?'

"He didn't win the race, but there was a point at which he was ahead. Here I was worried that he would be upset because he wasn't one of the winners; he focused on the one moment when he was in the lead."

- Tom: "Did you see my lead?"

MAGIC MOMENTS
CHART THE MILESTONES

Recovery was a long process; it did not just happen overnight. There were physical signs that let Jane know that her health was improving. Once again, it was her morning magic moments that helped her notice and chart her milestones.

"When I was really sick, I was in bed, and I couldn't do anything. One morning, I was well enough to get up and make crepes, to make breakfast for the boys.

"Before that, I sometimes felt that I had so much responsibility. Making meals was a chore. After realizing that I might have died, and never even be able to prepare food again, being able to do it seemed like a privilege."

- making breakfast for my boys

Friends took her to their cabin at Crystal Mountain.

"We went for long walks. I was aware of sounds, even the slightest noise in nature was a great joy to me."

- hearing the water gurgle in the creek

"It seemed like a miracle. I felt so lucky to be able to be there again and hear that."

WHY WRITE?

T. Stephen Balch, M.D., medical director at the Jacquelyn Mc-Clure Lupus Treatment Center in Atlanta, says, "People with lupus are not responsible for developing the disease, but they are responsible for the way they react to it. Attitudes, feelings, and thoughts have an impact on health. The wellness-oriented mind is one that chooses to see the world in a positive light."

Jane says, "Lupus is a stress-related disease—that is documented—and it can flare up and come back, but when you strengthen your own position, it gives you an inner strength.

"In my case, writing helped me heal for sure."

Jane's attitude of gratitude has had long-range ramifications.

"After I got over the worst of the disease, I am happier and more content than I have ever been. For me, writing ten magic moments a day was healing in the present moment, while I was writing them, and also had later value. Even now when I read them, it's uplifting and inspiring. What can I say? It makes me happy."

A devout Presbyterian, Jane felt like God was punishing her when her children were born with problems and when she got sick herself.

"I turned away from God, how could he do this? Through the process of healing and accepting and looking at the good, I found my way back to some kind of faith.

"I now see that there is a kind of perfection in how my boys were born, and a perfection in my illness: not that it was meant to be, but that every situation has some perfection in it."

Her bout with lupus is thankfully many years behind her, but Jane still pays attention to the little things in life. Her voice has a lighthearted lift, a laughter in it, when she tells me of a recent small event that brightened her day.

"I was substitute teaching at Forest Ridge High School, teaching French. I hadn't been there for awhile, so I didn't know any of the kids. I went in one day; the next day, I was there again. A girl came into the classroom, and when she saw me she said, 'Oh hi, I'm glad you're back.'

"Little things like that—so nice, so sweet. And good to remember. I added it to my morning list."

Dr. Balch concludes, "People who are living well with their lupus . . . understand that lupus is not their whole life, only part of it." He adds that that distinction can make the difference "between enjoying life versus simply surviving life."

As Jane puts it, "There are a million things right in the world; why focus on what's wrong?"

APPLY THIS

When your world is crashing around you, you might believe you have nothing to be happy about. Well, you could be happy that you could make breakfast this morning, you could be happy that there is a robin in your yard who got a worm.

Think you could come up with ten a day?

It could be the difference between merely surviving life, or enjoying it.

May you have the commitment
to heal what has hurt you,
to allow it to come close to you,
and in the end,
become one with you.

—A Gaelic blessing

Thanks and Ever Thanks

Thank you and a big, proud, Mama Bear hug for each of my children.

James, for keeping me grounded by his common sense, calming me down. He is a man who has set high standards for himself, and lives up to them. Thanks for your excellent design work, and great spur-of-the-moment barbecues.

Peter, for listening during our early morning breakfasts on the beach as I hammer out ideas; he is my bouncer, because I bounce topics off him, and he lets me run with them until they are used up. Thanks for your conscientious attention to detail and fastidious formatting.

Emily, for her strength and her pencil case, and her no-nonsense (but room for a lot of fun) approach to life, for her constancy, and keeping me on track. Emily always chooses the high road, and then stays the course. The wonder is she brings the rest of us willingly along with her, laughing all the way.

Katherine, for her wisdom, on-target insight, her deep spirituality, and her graciousness in letting me hang out and write in some of her own haunts. Now she gets paid to pull the shots she always did so well at home. Katherine inspired me by cutting her luxurious locks to give her hair to children who had none, reminding me that "Less is more."

Carolyn, Peter's wife, sweet and thoughtful and dedicated to family, I am blessed in such a daughter-in-love.

Cousin Annie Garde—whenever she breezes into town, my creativity quotient soars.

The baristas who greet me with a friendly smile and remember my drink (tall vanilla non-fat latte single shot dense foam with a twist of orange zest).

Mary Sandstrom, now at Top Pot Zeitgeist; Dan Reveles and Holly Odegard at Coffee Animals; Jamie Gentry, Scott, Kimberley Kevin, also a writer, JoAnn Baker, Carrie Pendleton, Chris McGonickle, Leslie Hunter, Lindsey Oftedahl, Emily McNaughten and Laurie Banek at Tully's.

And the friendly faces at Teahouse Kuan Yin, Celeste Dettmer, Duolan Li and James Labe. You may have wondered what I am writing to the wee hours; many the nights I closed the place at midnight or after.

For my Jesuit friends: Fr. Mike Bayard, S.J. gentle, humble, intelligent. Thanks for letting me be part of the Ignatian Silent Retreat and for teaching me so much by your own quiet example. Fr. Paul Janowiak, S.J., spent hours with me, and was the first to say, "You can do this," forcibly. Fr. Paul is a high-energy, impassioned orator; an author himself, he knows the hard work involved. Thanks for sharing Mary Oliver with me, and for being a good listener.

Elaine St. James's encouragement set me free to fly: "You are a writer, that's what you do. Do what you love."

Diane Wright, for questions that challenge me, a master of deadlines (how does she do it?), and the other "ladies" of the Uppity Ladies Book Club, writers and readers all.

Dorothy and Bill, stalwart and true; after all these years, they still stand by my side.

Shane Plossu, so busy telling others how wonderful they are, that he doesn't see, he is the wonderful one.

Beth Harrington, for fast typing, smiling cyberdrops, and diskette drivebys.

For those who spent time with me, exploring the topic of writing and healing, Dee Smith, Faye Anderson, Terry Copeland thanks to you.

Parker, I admire the work that you do with men in prison, healing the father-son wound through writing.

Erich Parce, thanks for keeping music alive in my life, and Melissa, as always, for being sweet and supportive.

Iris Corallo, popping in and pushing me to ride fast and far, goading me on, yet stopping to delight in the sunflowers, pick the blackberries, and drink free samples at the winery along the way.

Thanks to the Edmonds Library. Internet is there, but nothing beats a good reference librarian for tracking down the exactitude of an esoteric fact. Who coined the term "stream of consciousness"? How many acres are there in Central Park? Who was the first to say "attitude of gratitude"? Thanks to Evie Wilson-Lingbloom, Ginny Rollett, Cindy Lyons, Sunny Strong, and Tom Reynolds—they are like detectives. No matter how obtuse my request, they always come through with a smile.

Much gratitude to my editor, Marnie Cochran. We will forever associate this book with the coming of her daughter Katherine. Marnie, you are a great labor coach guiding to this book to life. If you want something done, ask a busy woman.

If Marnie is the labor coach, my agents, Jane Dystel and Miriam Goderich, are the gifted midwives, with a special talent—they've seen a lot of books born, but they make me feel like mine is the only one.

And a deep deep thanks, with much admiration, to those who so generously shared their stories and their writing. They did it to help others. Their lives are an example, an inspiration, and put me in awe at the resiliency of the human spirit.

Jan Eggebraaten, feisty and fun, with an open candor, stark honesty.

Lisa Hauser, lyric and tender, compassionate.

Jenna Buffaloe, adventurous and strong, invincible.

Jack Kennedy, brilliant and kind, his gentleness and wisdom set my heart on fire.

Tim Shields, a visionary and dreamer, determined and committed.

Patti Kajlich, warm and caring, willing to work things through.

Cassie, good natured and solid, like a rock.

Victoria Clearman, dedicated to truth, and to her family.

Leslie, a big heart in a little frame.

Debra Adams, tenacious and down-to-earth goodness.

Mike Reagan, expansive and artistic, patriotic and loyal.

Connie Sue Brown, creative and bright-hearted, vibrant.

Jane Koning, steady, with sense of wonder at the world.

And finally, to St. Ignatius of Loyola, my special friend in times of darkness and light.

Thanks to the human heart by which we live,
Thanks to its tenderness, its joys, and fears,
To me the meanest flower that blows can give
Thoughts that do often lie too deep for tears.

—William Wordsworth

Appendix

These are graphic examples of the problem-solving device discussed in Chapter 5, Edward De Bono's PMI. The P stands for Plus, the M is Minus, and the I, Interesting.

In the first case, a possible opening at a local community college teaching Medieval English came to my attention. I was not sure if I wanted to apply, or to continue my career as a writer and speaker.

First, I made the Provisional Decision to apply for the position. I did a PMI.

I will apply to teach Medieval English at Community College.

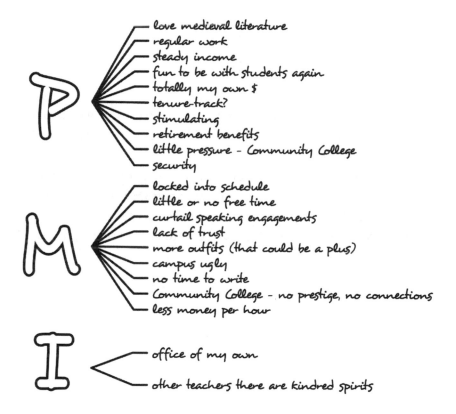

Then I took the opposite stance, framed just as definitely, and did a PMI on this alternate decision.

I will stay with Speaking/Writing.

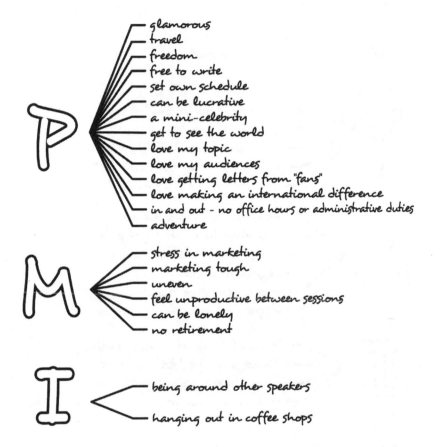

glamorous
travel
freedom
free to write
set own schedule
can be lucrative
a mini-celebrity
get to see the world
love my topic
love my audiences
love getting letters from "fans"
love making an international difference
in and out - no office hours or administrative duties
adventure

stress in marketing
marketing tough
uneven
feel unproductive between sessions
can be lonely
no retirement

being around other speakers
hanging out in coffee shops

It was not any one item, but rather the energy I got surrounding the second choice that made me decide firmly (and happily) not to apply for the teaching position and instead concentrate on building up my career as an author and professional speaker with books and presentations.

Sometimes one PMI is enough.

Recently, I was planning a trip to Cork, Ireland. While on hold for airline reservations, I debated whether to come back via Dublin, rather than go round-trip in and out of Cork. I made a snap decision and did a quick PMI.

I will return from Dublin instead of Cork

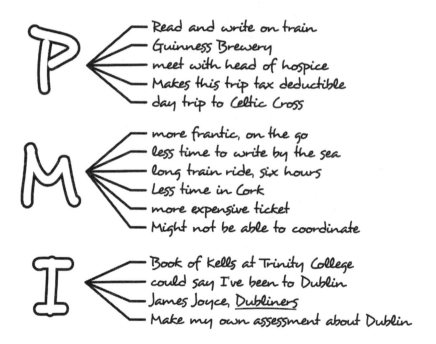

P
- Read and write on train
- Guinness Brewery
- meet with head of hospice
- Makes this trip tax deductible
- day trip to Celtic Cross

M
- more frantic, on the go
- less time to write by the sea
- long train ride, six hours
- Less time in Cork
- more expensive ticket
- Might not be able to coordinate

I
- Book of Kells at Trinity College
- could say I've been to Dublin
- James Joyce, Dubliners
- Make my own assessment about Dublin

By the time the reservation clerk came back on the line, I had made up my mind to see the Book of Kells, and to down a pint of stout at the Guinness Brewery.

Resources

Adams, Kathleen MA, LPC. *The Way of the Journal: A Journal Therapy Workbook for Healing.* 2d ed. Lutherville, MD: Sidran Press, 1998.

Bergan, Jacqueline Syrup, and S. Marie Schwan. *Freedom: A Guide for Prayer.* Take and Receive series. Winona, Minn.: Saint Mary's Press, 1988.

Cameron, Julia. *The Artist's Way: A Spiritual Path to Higher Creativity.* San Francisco: Tarcher, 1992.

Capacchione Lucia. *The Power of Your Other Hand: A Course in Channeling the Inner Wisdom of the Right Brain.* Rev. ed. Los Angeles, CA: New Page Books, 2001.

Conley-Weaver, Robyn. *What Really Matters to Me: A Guided Journal.* Cincinnati, Ohio: Walking Stick Press, 2001.

de Bono, Edward. *de Bono's Thinking Course.* Rev. ed. New York: Facts on File, 1994.

De Salvo, Louise. *Writing As a Way of Healing: How Telling Our Stories Transforms Our Lives.* San Francisco: HarperCollins, 1999.

Harris, Miriam Kalman, ed. *Rape, Incest, Battery: Women Writing Out the Pain.* Fort Worth, Texas: Texas Christian University Press, 2000.

Klauser, Henriette Anne. "To Write or Type?" *Personal Journaling,* December 2001.

_____. *Writing on Both Sides of the Brain.* San Francisco: Harper-Collins, 1987.

_____. *Put Your Heart on Paper.* New York: Bantam Books, 1996.

_____. *Write It Down, Make It Happen,* New York: Simon & Schuster, 2001.

Linn, Dennis, Sheila Fabricant Linn, and Matthew Linn, S.J. *Sleeping with Bread: Holding What Gives You Life.* Mahwah, N.J.: Paulist Press, 1995.

Matsakis, Aphrodite, Ph.D. *I Can't Get Over It: A Handbook for Trauma Survivors.* 2d ed. Oakland, CA: New Harbinger 1996.

Pennebaker, James W. *Opening Up: The Healing Power of Expressing Emotions.* Reprint. New York: Guilford Press, 1997.

Ramsland, Katherine. "Shelter from the Storm" (dealing with life-threatening illness), *Personal Journaling,* April 2001, p. 18.

Rich, Phil, and Stuart A. Copans. *The Healing Journey: Your Journal of Self-Discovery.* New York: John Wiley & Sons, 1998.

Richman, Linda. *I'd Rather Laugh: How to Be Happy Even When Life Has Other Plans for You.* New York: Warner Books, 2002.

SARK. *Eat Mangoes Naked, Finding Pleasure Everywhere and Dancing with the Pits.* New York: Fireside, 2001.

Selling, Bernard. *Writing from Within, A Guide to Creativity and Life Story Writing.* 3d ed. Claremont, CA: Hunter House, 1988–98.

About the Author

Henriette Anne Klauser, Ph.D. is the author of *Writing on Both Sides of the Brain, Put Your Heart on Paper*, and *Write It Down/Make It Happen.* Dr. Klauser is the president of Writing Resources, a seminar and consulting organization in existence since 1979 with offices in Edmonds, Washington. She has taught at the University of Washington, California State University, Seattle University, University of Lethbridge (Canada), and Fordham University. Her clients include Fortune 500 companies, government agencies, universities, and national associations thoughtout North America. A past trustee of the Pacific Northwest Writers Conference, she is listed in the International Who's Who in Business and Professional Women. Her workshops have taken her around the world, including to London, England; Cairo, Egypt and the island of Skyros in Greece.

Henriette has a special devotion to St. Ignatius of Loyola, and like him, she carries a small notebook with her wherever she goes. She personally reads every letter she receives and loves getting mail from her readers.

You may contact her at: Henriette Anne Klauser, Ph.D.
Writing Resources
P. O. Box 1555
Edmonds, WA 98020
USA

Or email: henriette@henrietteklauser.com

Website: www.henrietteklauser.com